AN INT   THE:
POLICY, PLA   FINANCING

WITHDRAWN

21/4/23

Consultant Editor: Jo Campling

An Introduction to Health: Policy, Planning and Financing

Brian Abel-Smith

LONGMAN
London and New York

Longman Group Limited
Longman House, Burnt Mill,
Harlow, Essex CM20 2JE, England
and Associated Companies throughout the world

*Published in the United States of America
by Longman Publishing, New York*

First published 1994

ISBN 0 582 23866 8 CSD
ISBN 0 582 23865 X PPR

British Library Cataloguing-in-Publication Data

A catalogue record for this book is
available from the British Library

Library of Congress Cataloging-in-Publication Data

Abel-Smith, Brian.
  An introduction to health : policy, planning, and financing /
Brian Abel-Smith
    p.   cm.
  Includes bibliographical references and index.
  ISBN 0-582-23866-8. -- ISBN 0-582-23865-X (pbk.)
    1. Health planning.   2. Medical care--Finance--Government policy.
I. Title.
RA394.9.A24   1994
362.1--dc20   94-7222
                                                                  CIP

Set by 7 00 in Times
Produced by Longman Singapore Publishers (Pte) Ltd.
Printed in Singapore

CONTENTS

PREFACE

This book is about how to improve health in a cost-effective and politically acceptable way. It is not just about health services as they are not the most important determinant of health improvement. But they are an area where extra money can be spent to limited advantage, thus restricting the money available to improve health in other ways.

The book covers policy, planning and financing as they are so closely interrelated, and it does so in the contexts of both developed and developing countries. Much has been written about the use of this last term. It has been said to be insulting and patronising to describe countries as 'developing'. But this terminology is used here, partly because it is in common use and partly because there is no satisfactory alternative. The term 'Third World' is no longer appropriate now that the 'Second World' is likely to be divided between the first and third, and the term 'South' is clearly geographically incorrect.

The focus is on the policy aspects of planning rather than on planning techniques which are covered elsewhere (e.g. Green 1992).[1] The issue of finance is given prominence, as over the last ten years it has seemed to governments in both developed and developing countries to be a central, if not the central, political issue in planning for health. Money spent in one way cannot be spent in another. In developed countries the problem presents itself in the guise of containing the cost of health care, whether the bulk of it is in the private sector or the public sector. In some developing countries the problem presents itself as how to maintain present health spending, let alone find more money to move towards the objectives endorsed by governments when the World Health Organisation's 'Health For All' initiative was presented in 1977.

The book deals with both developed and developing countries on the grounds that each has lessons applicable to the other. Moreover, the problem is essentially the same: how to spend money most effectively on health development. The lessons from the developed countries come from long historical experience and better data and demonstrate what can go wrong as well as what can go right. Those from the developing countries result from having meagre resources, and so being under much stronger pressure to find ways of promoting health which the countries can afford. Moreover the hard distinction between developed and developing countries conceals the facts that there are large groups of affluent persons in most developing countries whose health problems are similar to those of the developed countries and that there are large variations in the income and demographic situation of different developing countries.

The book does not pretend to be value-free. It starts from the value premises underlying the 'Health for All' programme. The premises are that all people have a right to health, in so far as this can be achieved. It follows from this that the aim of equity between countries, regions and individuals should underlie health policies. The book draws considerably on health economics and other social sciences. But it is deliberately written to demystify – to explain economic concepts in simple terms so that, for example, trained health personnel can readily understand the arguments.

The book is divided into four parts. The first deals with the major determinants of health and health policy in its broadest sense. The second narrows the perspective to health service planning and the third to health service financing. The final part concentrates on how to create both efficient and user-friendly health services.

The author wishes to thank Lucy Gilson, Julian Le Grand and Anne Mills, all of whom were kind enough to read a draft of the book and make valuable comments and suggestions which I have greedily used to improve what I have written. The faults that remain in the book should be attributed to my own obstinacy or stupidity in failing to take their good advice.

Brian Abel-Smith

Notes

1 See, for example, Green, A. (1992) *An Introduction to Health Planning in Developing Countries*, Oxford University Press, Oxford.

PART ONE

The determinants of health

CHAPTER 1

Introduction

Over the past 150 years, the expectation of life for human beings in nearly all parts of the world has been transformed. This has been particularly marked in the industrialised countries towards the North of the world where about 30 years or more has been added to an average expectation of life of about 40 years for men and 45 for women. Some developing countries have made similar or very substantial progress since the Second World War, for example China, Costa Rica, Singapore, South Korea, Sri Lanka and Taiwan. While some exceptional groups of population in remote parts of Latin America or North India may have had a long expectation of life much earlier, this represents a transformation in whole countries compared to their whole past history in so far as it is known.

Why has this occurred? What determines the health of populations? This simple but critical question is by no means easy to answer. This is surprising in view of the vast expenditure on health research over the twentieth century and particularly in the later part of it. This is because the investment in health research has been largely biomedical – how to improve the treatment of particular diseases in individuals rather than how to improve the health of whole populations. As a result, a vast amount is known about disease but far too little about health. Two to four hundred years ago, a much higher proportion of writing about health in the English language concentrated on health in general than does writing in the past 50 years. However, in the past 20 years the issue of the health of whole populations has at last begun to be given somewhat greater prominence.

The essential question which needs to be answered is why the populations of some countries appear to be healthier than others. Or to narrow the question why do people live longer in some countries than others? Is it because they have more health services or better health services than others or is it from other causes? The same questions need to be asked within countries. Why do some groups in society not only live longer than others in the same country but appear to have less illness and less disability? The groups may be based on geographical parts of the country, on sex, on occupation, on income group, on racial origin, or on other criteria. But before these questions can be approached, we need to be clear about what we mean by health. One cannot say that one population or group is healthier than another unless there is some reliable way of measuring it.

The meaning of health

In its constitution of 1948, the World Health Organisation defined health as 'A state of complete physical, mental and social well-being and not merely the absence of disease or infirmity'.

This expresses high rhetorical ideals but it gives no indication of how health can be measured. What is physical well-being and who is to determine it – the patient or the doctor? How can mental well-being be measured let alone social well-being? The Health for All strategy of 1981 seemed a bit more precise when it talked of the aim of maximising economic and social life. But how does one measure ability to work as distinct from the fact of working? Are the tasks of child care or housework part of 'economic' life, even though there is no payment for them?

Such health statistics as there are, which can be compared between countries, measure ill-health rather than health. The only really reliable statistics are of death in those countries where deaths are accurately recorded and the age of the deceased person is known. Death is a fact though there has been some debate about how it should be determined. The concept of morbidity is much more difficult. At first sight it may seem possible to use the number of cases presented to doctors or hospitals where the doctor can find clinical evidence of ill-health. But there are three snags. First, there are many conditions which are very real to the patient but for which clinical evidence is lacking, such as back pain or almost any form of mental illness. Second, in all societies, by no means all health problems lead to a visit to a doctor. Most cases of ill-health are treated by self-care and family care, with or without a visit to a pharmacist. Some cases go to alternative healers under a variety of labels in developed countries and what is often just called 'traditional medicine' in developing countries can also have great variety. Third, feeling unwell is not the only reason for going to the doctor. If time off work on full pay or half pay depends on a certificate of incapacity to work issued by a doctor, then inevitably there will be some who simply want to sleep in after a late night or take a paid holiday to attend a wedding or a football match. As the British Medical Association once put it frankly, 'in most cases the doctor does no more than countersign the patient's declaration of his fitness or not to work'[1].

Does one then assess ill-health by questioning the patient? One approach is to ask about restricted activity. Did the person go to work or school or do the housework as usual? Was the person at home all day because of illness? Was the person in bed because of illness? A second approach is to ask more positively about what the patient is able to do – climb stairs, walk a mile, run for a bus, peel potatoes, and so on. A third approach is to ask about short term and long-standing illnesses. A fourth is to ask about perceived health: 'Would you say that your health was very good, good, moderate, poor, or very poor?'.

The trouble is that such questions are likely to be answered in terms of people's reference groups, such as other members of the family, neighbours, work mates. Thus people living in a mining village, where most men have some lung condition, are likely to judge on different criteria from those living in leafy, unpolluted suburbs. A particular danger is that the reference group is likely to be taken from one's own social class. Expectations of health are likely to differ not only between countries but within countries.

One must conclude that the concept of health is elusive. This is particularly the case as it has different dimensions. Mildred Blaxter lists five: disease, disability, frequency of illness, malaise (tiredness, depression, trouble with nerves, sleeplessness and worry) and fitness (Blaxter 1985: pp. 131–71)[2]. It is hard to see how these five dimensions could ever be added together in any meaningful way. And their relative importance would differ between developed and developing countries because of the different pattern of disease.

There can hardly be only one measuring rod. Different measures may be useful for different purposes. The easiest measure is mortality and this is correlated with morbidity over a wide area. But there are conditions, such as asthma, which people should never die of. And mortality has little connection with mental illness. It is extremely difficult to say whether people have more mental illness today than a century ago. Of course more cases are presented to doctors and hospitals, but is this a useful measure? It is easy to romanticise the life of an agricultural village whether in Europe a century ago or in Africa or Asia today. One can depict it as a low-pace life full of neighbour-liness and lacking in stress. Alternatively one can depict it as a life of constant uncertainty about subsistence, ruled by the weather and regulated by very strong social controls. What social and economic environment really is conducive to mental well-being? And how far is it affected by religious beliefs and practices?

Approaches to examining the fundamental determinants of health

There are two different approaches to trying to ascertain the fundamental determinants of health and their relative importance. The first is historical. What changes took place in particular societies which had a large improvement in mortality rates and which might have caused the improvement? The second approach is comparative. What are the differences between countries or regions with good and bad mortality rates which might explain the difference?

The historical approach

Britain is the country with the oldest reliable set of statistics. This is because registration of deaths by cause was introduced as early as

1837 (Flinn 1966: p. 14)[3]. When the process of extending expectation of life is examined, two important conclusions emerge. First, the major reductions in mortality have been at the earlier ages. In 1851, mortality rates were about 20 times higher at ages 1 to 14 than in 1981, about ten times higher at ages 15 to 44 and only twice as high at ages 55 to 64. The extension of life beyond age 65 has been relatively small. Second, Mckeown showed that the decline in mortality between 1851 and 1900 was entirely due to the reduction in death from infectious disease (Mckeown 1965: p. 42)[4]. Five groups of diseases accounted for the decline from 1838 onwards – tuberculosis for a little less than half; typhus, typhoid and fever for about a fifth; cholera and dysentery for nearly a tenth; and smallpox for a twentieth (Mckeown 1965: p. 57)[5].

Why did this occur? Was it because the ratio of doctors to the population increased? In 1851 there was already one doctor to less than a thousand population (Loudon 1986: p. 215)[6]: the ratio was much the same in 1931 though medical education had changed beyond recognition. Was it because hospitals were developed which cared for those with infectious disease? Before 1867, the poor with infectious diseases were admitted to workhouses where they were 'treated' or at least isolated. This was because nearly all the charitable hospitals deliberately refused to admit 'fever' cases through fear of cross-infection. After 1867 a rapid building programme was started to provide public hospitals for fever cases in London: a special health authority ('the Metropolitan Asylums Board') was created to deal with the problem (Ayers 1971)[7]. Over 6,000 beds were built. In the next 32 years some 10,000 persons with infectious diseases died in these isolation hospitals, but in the same period over 95 per cent of deaths from the principal zymotic diseases occurred outside them (Ayers 1971: pp. 120–3)[8]. Thus the development was too little and too late.

Was the change due to developments in medical knowledge? How far could doctors cure people with infectious diseases? The introduction of sulphonamides in the 1930s may have helped to reduce deaths from bronchitis, whooping cough, measles, scarlet fever and puerperal fever in maternity cases. But apart from the diphtheria antitoxin developed in 1894, little could be claimed for cure until the antibiotics became available for civilian use from 1945 and streptomycin for tuberculosis from 1947. This was after the major reduction in mortality had occurred (Mckeown 1979: pp. 50–4)[9]. Was it because of specific preventive actions? Smallpox vaccination dates from 1798 but it was not widely used until the late nineteenth century. Immunisation for diphtheria and whooping cough did not come until the 1940s, for typhoid and measles until the 1950s and for polio-myelitis until the 1950s. Again this was long after the major reductions in mortality had occurred.

Was it because of personal hygiene? Soap was considered a luxury in the early nineteenth century and was taxed accordingly. As late as 1855 it would cost a working man about one tenth of his weekly income to buy a bar of soap. What effect was the abolition of this luxury tax likely to have had? There would have been an effect on the incidence of typhus but not much else (Mckeown 1979: p. 59)[10]. Was it because of the introduction of safe water and sanitation – the massive municipal programme increasingly undertaken following Chadwick's 1842 Report on the Sanitary Condition of the Labouring Population? For example, between 1858 and 1865, 80 miles of sewers were installed in London alone (Open University 1985: p. 54)[11]. The task was largely completed in all urban areas by the end of the century. This was undoubtedly very important for cholera and typhoid but would have had little impact on measles, whooping cough, diphtheria or tuberculosis. Mckeown suggests that the efforts of the sanitary reformers were only responsible for about a quarter of the decline in mortality (1979: p. 54)[12]. Particularly striking was the fact that deaths from tuberculosis were falling by about 10 per cent a year from 1871 onwards without any specific measure of prevention or cure.

Mckeown reached the conclusion that the major factor, other than water and sanitation, accounting for about half the decline in mortality, was improvements in living standards and particularly in nutrition. This was partly due to declining family size and partly due to lower food prices which in turn were due to improvements in cultivated land, yields per acre, and later the technology which enabled food to be imported cheaply in the new metal ships paid for by manufactured goods (Mckeown 1979: p. 54)[13]. This is consistent with the fact that France had much lower real wages in the nineteenth century and much higher tuberculosis mortality than Britain (Barnes 1992)[14].

While this conclusion is very important, it raises many further questions. What was the relative importance of calories, protein and vitamins? Did the improvements in living standards reach the very poor – particularly widows and their young children? What were the urban and rural differences? Were there also reductions in the physical energy needed for work and daily life? Was the factory environment also improving? Is this the whole story?

Recent work by Szreter (1988: pp. 1–38)[15] has examined particular periods to see how far they fit in with the above generalisation. Between 1820 and 1870 real wages fell but there was little change in overall mortality rates: indeed they became worse in urban areas, though better in rural areas. This difference was probably due to the effects of rapid urbanisation and industrialisation. The improvement was, however, noticeable between 1870 and 1900 soon after London's main sewers were complete and clean water was available, with these developments spreading to the provinces in this 30-year period.

Infant mortality remained at around 150 per thousand in the early years of the twentieth century before starting to decline despite lower real wages. Infantile diarrhoea increased its incidence in the 1890s and became a principal cause of death in the first year of life. The first decade of the twentieth century was the period when the first generation of literate women became mothers; virtually all of them could read or write as a result of compulsory education enacted from 1881. Literacy gave women access to new information about health (Williams 1986: p. 391)[16]. It was also the period when infant welfare centres were developed, originally by women volunteers, to monitor the growth of infants and educate mothers in child care. By the mid-1920s there was a country-wide network of centres. From 1918, local authorities were authorised to provide salaried midwives and health visitors as well as infant welfare centres, and in time the child health services became professionalised and increasingly included visits to mothers of new-born children in their own homes (Williams 1986: p. 391)[17]. In the same period, there was active concern about slum housing, with again local authorities starting to intervene. Another relevant factor is the availability of sterilised milk. It was not until about 1930 that milk supplies became safe (Atkins 1992: pp. 207–28)[18].

Anne Oakley has shown that in the interwar period, maternal mortality obstinately refused to be reduced by the introduction of antenatal care but only finally responded with the improvements in living standards, full employment, greater equality and food rationing that came with the Second World War (Oakley 1984: pp. 87–115)[19].

But even if Mckeown's broad thesis of the major importance of nutrition and living standards is accepted, it does not follow that economic growth inevitably improves health standards. It can lead to factors adverse to health as well as factors which favour it. With greater affluence has come the increase in the consumption of alcohol and, until recently, tobacco. It has brought the heavy toll of motor accidents, the excessive use of drugs, the decline in physical activity, the introduction of a large range of new chemical substances with unknown consequences and adverse changes in diet (greater consumption of sugar and animal fats and decline in the consumption of coarse root vegetables and rough bread). Thus while infectious diseases have declined, there has been a rise in the incidence of the diseases which are associated with more affluent societies even though those diseases strike the poor more than the rich. The same is happening to the more affluent in developing countries.

Variations among developed countries

While Mckeown has attempted to explain the very broad trend of mortality among what are now the developed countries, his theory does not attempt to explain the large differences in the expectation of life among developed countries. Why, for example have both sexes in

Japan the highest life expectancy in the world? Why is Iceland the runner-up for female life expectancy? Why do Southern European countries have much higher expectation of life than would be expected for their level of living? One possible explanation is diet – the prevalence of fish eating in Iceland and Japan and the extensive use of vegetable fats, rather than animal fats, in Southern Europe. Nor does the thesis account satisfactorily for the wide differences in expectation of life among developed countries with similar levels of living.

Correlations with standardised mortality among the majority of developed countries in the OECD, for which data were available, showed some suggestive results (Matsaganis 1992)[20]. Higher income countries tend to have lower mortality rates, but this may be due to the fact that these countries spend more on education. But there is evidence to suggest that the impact of income on health gradually declines as countries move from lower to higher levels of income. Moreover, the more unequal the distribution of income within a country the greater the inequalities in health. Higher mortality rates were also found in countries where urban pollution was worse. There was also found to be significantly higher mortality, the higher the consumption of animal fats. Less clear was the association with cigarette consumption measured 15 years earlier as the effects take time to develop. There was no clear significant association with mortality of urbanisation, hospital bed provision or alcohol consumption. Differences in mortality have little to do with the provision of medical care, though the latter may improve the quality if not the quantity of life. Thus later findings confirm the conclusion of Archie Cochrane and his colleagues made in 1978 that 'health service factors are relatively unimportant in explaining the differences in mortality between developed countries' (Cochrane *et al.* 1978: pp. 200–5)[21].

Correlations between countries suggested that infant mortality tended to be higher where the distribution of income was more unequal. This was particularly the case with females. Environmental pollution seemed also to be linked to infant mortality but not as strongly as with overall mortality. On the other hand infant mortality seemed to be higher where the consumption of animal fats was lower. Turning to causes of death, cancers seemed to be linked to education levels: there was less cancer where they were higher, but education levels are also associated with income levels. There was more cancer mortality in countries with large proportions of people living in urban areas. Not surprisingly greater cigarette smoking was linked to greater cancer mortality but this was not true of alcohol consumption. In the case of cardiovascular diseases, greater animal fat consumption seemed to result in more deaths from this cause. Mortality from respiratory diseases tended to rise as income, doctor provision, and alcohol consumption fell, and rise as urbanisation increased.[22]

Variations among developing countries

How far is the historical experience of Europe relevant to health development in the developing countries today? The developing countries have different economic and social structures to those of nineteenth-century Europe. Moreover, technological developments in medicine, both in prevention and cure, have led to a number of specific interventions which are effective and cheap and which were not available a century ago. Nevertheless, Mckeown's analysis does make one question whether developing countries are wise to spend a half or more of their health resources on hospitals when about a third of the population of East Asia and a quarter of the population of Africa lacks sufficient protein and even urban provision of safe water and sanitation is far from adequate.

Economic growth as measured by gross national product per head does not mean that a developing country is necessarily improving its nutrition standards. The modern sector may be outbidding the rural population for the limited food supplies. An emphasis on export crops can reduce the land available for growing traditional foods. The movement of population, particularly towards the cities can lead to the spread of infectious diseases and the formidable problems of providing water and sanitation as cities grow and shanty towns surround them (Cumper 1985: pp. 29–31)[23]. Accompanying this may be the pollution caused by motor vehicles and factories. Even irrigation projects, if their health consequences are neglected, can lead to worse health problems such as schistosomiasis. Finally economic growth can lead to more income inequality between income groups, rural and urban areas, worse distribution of food within the family as women lose control of the food supply, and the growth of cigarette smoking and consumption of alcohol.

In the middle 1980s, the Rockefeller Foundation selected five regions that were outliers in the sense that they appeared to have much higher expectation of life than would be expected from their level of living and commissioned studies of their health development (Halstead *et al.* 1987)[24]. They were China, Costa Rica, Cuba, Kerala State in India and Sri Lanka. The study of Cuba was not however completed. The infant mortality rate, expectation of life and income per head in US dollars of four of these countries are shown in Table 1.1. Some of the features of these selected countries are shown in Table 1.2.

The common features of the countries identified were a heavy emphasis on nutrition, at least some land reform, very well-developed primary education which covered females, above average equality of income, priority given to health and community participation and quite well-developed rural health care. But some of these characteristics cannot readily be quantified.

Another detailed study has been made of two states in India – Kerala and West Bengal. The latter is substantially richer and at first

Table 1.1 **The success stories among developing countries**

	Infant mortality rate	Expectation of life (years)	Income per head (US dollars)
Costa Rica	21	73	1430
Cuba	20	75	1000*
Sri Lanka	34	69	320
China**	13–22	69	310

*estimated
** based on incomplete data
Source: Author' s summary from Halstead *et al.* 1987, pp. 14, 95, 126, 160.

Table 1.2 **Factors influencing health**

	China	Sri Lanka	Cuba	Costa Rica
Food policy	Food for work	Food subsidies	Food subsidies	School meals, food for vulnerable groups
Land reform	Yes	Partial	Yes	Partial
Greater equality of income	Yes	Yes	Yes	Yes
Enrolment in primary education				
1960	70–80	100	70–80	100
1980	100	100	100	100
Water				
urban	50%	65%	?	95%
rural	40%	18%	?	68%
Sanitation				
urban	?	80%	?	43%
rural	?	63%	?	82%
Rural health coverage	Uneven	Average	Very good	Very good
Emphasis on participation	Yes	Some	Yes	Yes
Political priority for health	Yes	Above average	Yes	Yes

Source: Author's summary from Halstead *et al.* 1987, pp. 176, 192, 203.

sight some of the findings seem to contradict the above (see Table 1.3).

Both the expectation of life and the infant mortality rate are much better in Kerala. But nutrition is better in West Bengal, though there has been some dispute about the evidence for this, and there is much more piped water in West Bengal. On the other hand, income inequality is less in Kerala and the education system aims, as a minimum, to give all children a primary education. Educational priorities in West Bengal are more meritocratic: it has a considerably lower rate

Table 1.3   **The comparison of Kerala and West Bengal**

	Kerala	West Bengal
Expectation of Life		
male	59	49
female	59	51
Infant Mortality (1970)		
urban	40	61
rural	56	113
Per head GDP (Rupees 1975–6)	1000	1100
Calorie intake		
rural (1972–6)	1983	2279
urban (1971–2)	2103	2431
Protein intake	Lower	Higher
Piped water and sanitation	Lower	Higher but poorly maintained
Industrialisation	Low and falling	High and rising
Literacy (1971)	60%	35%
Female education (1978)		
age 6–10	86%	58%
age 11–13	74%	32%
Water	Boiled	Not boiled
Income equality		
Gini coefficient 1973–4	0.32	0.30
Voting (1960)	84%	56%

Source: Author's summary from Nag, M., 'The impact of social and economic development on mortality' in Halstead *et al.* 1987, pp. 57–77.

of attendance at primary education but a much greater development of secondary education. Kerala may well correct for the lack of piped water by the widespread habit of boiling water before use. Participation in elections is much higher in Kerala which has long had a high proportion of population who are Christian. While again some of these factors are difficult to quantify, it does appear that the effects of a low average income per head can be offset by other factors which are favourable to health.

The study focuses attention on three further factors. Average income per head is a poor indicator. What is important is the distribution of income, as this is likely to affect the poorest people. Second, behaviour, in this case boiling water, can apparently be significant. Third, education and particularly female education is an important variable to which too little attention has been given in the past. It was almost entirely neglected by Mckeown. Compulsory education in Britain dates from 1881, and by the turn of the century mothers had at least primary education. This may have made them more responsive to the messages of trained midwives and health visitors.

A further outlier is Tanzania. Though it is among the poorest African countries, it has the third lowest infant mortality for sub-Saharan Africa. By the early 1980s, it had 98 per cent school enrolment at the primary stage with 95 per cent female enrolment. By the end of the 1970s, 70 per cent of the population was within 5 kilometres of a health institution. Where the health situation was below the regional average, this was associated with lower maternal literacy, poorer water supply and lower levels of immunisation (WHO 1976: p. 36)[25].

Female education

A study of 99 developing countries showed that poor countries which have given priority to investments in education have lower infant mortality rates and longer expectations of life than countries with less educated populations and much higher per capita income. Trends in 13 African countries between 1975 and 1985 show that a 10 per cent increase in female literacy reduces child mortality by 10 per cent while changes in male literacy have little effect on child mortality (WHO 1976: p. 27)[26]. Surveys in 25 developing countries show that even one to three years of maternal schooling is enough to reduce child mortality by about 15 per cent, whereas similar paternal schooling achieves only a 6 per cent reduction (World Bank 1993: p. 42)[27]. Child survival rates in 1983 corresponded more closely to female enrolment in primary education in 1960 than to male enrolment (WHO 1976: pp. 75–8)[28]. There was thus a time lag for these women to enter child-bearing age.

Education improves a woman's capacity for self-care and maintenance of good health during pregnancy: it enables her to acquire greater knowledge and learn better child care practices. Education gives her confidence and the receptivity to benefit from child care services and understand the advice given by trained personnel.

The role of primary health care

The emphasis given to income and its distribution, to water, sanitation, education and lifestyle could imply that health care is of negligible importance. In fact the more health care is provided, the more morbidity comes to light. However, a study of ten primary care projects which could be evaluated led to the conclusion that 'well-designed and carefully implemented interventions can reduce infant and child mortality by as much as one half within five years at a cost below two per cent of per capita income' (Gwatkin *et al.* 1980)[29]. A particular case is Costa Rica where primary health care was gradually introduced to rural counties according to the demands of the inhabitants and their willingness to provide premises. This provided valuable controls in the form of those counties not yet having primary health care. In Table 1.4, there is clear evidence of improvements in the infant mortality rate as primary health care was extended, compared to those counties where it was not yet provided.

*Table 1.4   **Gain in life expectancy 1970–2 to 1974–6 in Costa Rica (Analysis by county)***

Coverage of rural health programme	Gain in years of life expectancy	Number of years the programme in effect	Gain in years of life expectancy
None	2.40	None	2.40
Under 25%	2.40	Under one year	4.21
25–49%	3.50	1 year under 2	4.48
50–74%	4.04	2 year under 3	3.41
Over 75%	5.07	3 year plus	5.06

Source: Saenz, L., 'Health changes during a decade: the Costa Rica case', in Halstead *et al.* 1987, pp. 143–4.

The longer the programme had been provided, the greater the improvement in expectation of life. Multiple correlation analysis suggests that 73 per cent of the fall in the infant mortality rate could be attributed to health programmes and 41 per cent of the decline to primary health care (see Table 1.5).

The demographic transition

When the health status of countries at different levels of development is examined, it appears that countries seem to go through three stages

Table 1.5 **Factors in the decline in infant mortality rates in Costa Rica (1972–80)**

	Percentages
Socio-economic progress	22
Fertility reduction	5
Secondary care	32
Primary care	41
TOTAL	100

Source: Rosero-Bixby, L., 'Infant mortality decline in Costa Rica', in Halstead *et al.* 1987, p. 136.

of health development (Frenk *et al.* 1991: pp. 21–38)[30]. The low income countries have the characteristics of high morbidity and high premature mortality, in both cases mainly from infectious diseases. The middle income countries have much lower mortality from infectious diseases but still a high morbidity from a similar pattern of diseases. What has changed is that these diseases do not lead to the same level of mortality. With the decline in infectious diseases there is generally a decline in fertility. The average age of the population increases both because of a decline in mortality at younger ages and because of the decline in fertility. The high income countries have much lower mortality from infectious diseases. Accidents, suicide and parasuicide become major causes of death in the 16 to 25 age group for males. In late middle age the major causes of mortality become diseases of the circulatory system, cardiovascular diseases and cancer. Among the old the degenerative diseases of the aged play an important role in mortality. The morbidity pattern is also different. The role of emotional and stress problems becomes important. Classifying countries into these three groups does, however, distort the picture as some countries contain regions with similarities to the first stage and other more affluent regions with similarities to the third stage of health development.

The demographic effects are the transition from a society with a very high proportion of children to a society with a high proportion of the population in middle and old age. One effect of the transition is, hopefully, a reduction of the birth rate. In many developed countries, it has fallen to below the level needed to maintain the number of the population in the long run. But it does not inevitably follow that better child survival will lower the birth rate. There is, as yet, little sign of this happening in most countries of sub-Saharan Africa. Nor has it happened in Jordan despite rapid economic growth. Thus countries can be faced with what has been called the 'demographic trap' (King 1990: pp. 664–7)[31] – high birth rate, low mortality rates of children and insufficient increases in income to raise average living standards. Such is the situation of Bangladesh which faces the prospect, in a generation' s time, of a population as large as that of the United States with a land area no larger than the State of North Carolina (Potts 1993: p. 10)[32]. Rapid population growth, without corresponding economic growth, cannot only lead to declining income per head but also to reduced ability of the country to finance education, health services and the spread of safe water and sanitation.

The interrelationships of the different factors

The attempt to isolate factors which are favourable to health is useful for analytical purposes but only tells part of the story. Factors do not operate in isolation from one another. The impact of two favourable factors together may well be much greater than the impact of each factor analysed separately. In other words, factors favourable to health may have a cumulative impact on health improvement. Nor is it possible to isolate factors which are inevitably to some extent interconnected. As a country becomes richer it can more readily find the money through taxes to finance better services, while still leaving in people's hands adequate money for food, housing and personal hygiene. On the other hand, better health contributes to economic growth. The economic potential of a country is clearly reduced if a high proportion of children suffer from stunted growth, there is a high rate of disablement, and about a tenth of the life of an average person is seriously disrupted by disease. Economic growth is not just the consequence of past physical investments but also of investments in people. The improved nutrition and health of new cohorts of workers should enable them to achieve higher productivity.

Conclusion

The developing countries face a somewhat different situation to that experienced by the countries that industrialised earlier. Many are in tropical or subtropical areas. More is now known about the means of controlling disease. The developing countries which have secured marked health improvement have achieved this by a decline in infectious diseases. This is despite the fact that food availability has been declining in Africa and not improving in South America. There has moreover been no significant reduction in fertility in Africa, Western Asia or parts of Latin America and progress with water and sanitation has been limited (Mckeown 1990: pp. 408–16)[33]. Increasing income for the poor would be likely to do most to improve health in these countries as the poor would be able to buy more food, better housing and better health care (World Bank 1993: p. 7)[34]. Second to this, education for women is of critical importance. In developed countries the average level of income becomes a less clear predictor of average levels of health but the extent of income inequality is still important.

There is a need for more studies of health development in different countries to see how far the factors listed above stand up to examination on larger sets of data. But the complex interrelationships between cause and effect make it difficult to estimate the relative importance of different factors.

Notes

1   Quoted in HMSO (1973), *Report of the Committee on Abuse of Social Security Benefits*, Cmnd. 5228, p. 66.
2   Blaxter, M. (1985), 'Self-definition of health status and consulting rates in primary care', *Quarterly Journal of Socal Affairs*, vol. 1, no. 2.
3   Flinn, M.W. (1966), *Report on the Sanitary Condition of the Labouring Population of Great Britain,* Edinburgh University Press, Edinburgh.
4   Mckeown, T. (1965), *Medicine in Modern Society*, Allen and Unwin, London, p. 42.
5   Mckeown (1965), *Medicine in Modern Society*.
6   Loudon, I. (1986), *Medical Care and the General Practitioner 1750–1850*, Clarendon, Oxford.
7   Ayers, G.M. (1971), *England's First State Hospitals 1867–1930*, Wellcome Institute, London.
8   Ayers (1971), *England's First State Hospitals*.
9   Mckeown, T. (1979), *The Role of Modern Medicine*, Blackwell, Oxford.
10   Kckeown (1979), *The Role of Modern Medicine*.
11   Open University (1985), *Caring for Health: History and Diversity*, Open University Press, Milton Keynes.
12   Mckeown (1979), *The Role of Modern Medicine*.
13   Mckeown (1979), *The Role of Modern Medicine*.
14   Barnes, D.S. (1992), 'The rise and fall of tuberculosis in Belle Epoque France', *Social History of Medicine*, vol. 5, no. 2.
15   Szreter, S. (1988), The importance of social intervention in Britain's mortality decline (1850–1914); a reinterpretation of the role of public health', *Social History of Medicine*, vol. 1, no. 1.
16   Williams, G. (1986), 'Save the babies', *World Health Forum*, vol. 7.
17   Williams (1986), 'Save the babies'.
18   Atkins, P.J. (1992), 'White poison?: the social consequences of milk consumption in London 1850–1939', *Social History of Medicine*, vol. 5, no. 2.
19   Oakley, A. (1984), *The Captured Womb*, Blackwell, Oxford.
20   Matsaganis, M. (1992), 'An economic approach to international and inter-regional mortality variations with special reference to Greece' (unpublished Ph.D thesis, University of Bristol).
21   Cochrane, A.L. *et al.* (1978), 'Health service input and mortality output in developed countries', *Journal of Epidemiology and Community Health*, no. 32.

22   For the findings quoted in this paragraph see Matsaganis (1992), *An Economic Approach.*

23   Cumper, G. (1985), 'Economic development, health services and health' in Lee, K. and Mills, A. (eds.), *The Economics of Health in Developing Countries*, Oxford.

24   Halstead, S.B., *et al.* (1987), *Good Health at Low Cost*, Rockefeller Foundation, New York.

25   World Health Organisation (1976), *Intersectoral Action for Health,* WHO, Geneva.

26   World Health Organisation (WHO) (1976), *Intersectoral Action.*

27   World Bank (1993), *World Development Report 1993: Issues in Health*, World Bank, Washington DC.

28   WHO (1976), *Intersectoral Action.*

29   Gwatkin, D.R., *et al.* (1980), *Can health and nutrition interventions make a difference?,* Overseas Development Monograph, no. 13.

30   Frenk, J., *et al.* (1991), 'Elements for a theory of the health transition', *Health Transition Review*, vol. 1, no.1.

31   King, M. (1990), 'Health in a sustainable state', *Lancet*, 15.

32   Potts, M. (1993), 'Family planning, demography and safe motherhood', *News on Health Care in Developing Countries*, Uppsala, Sweden, no. 1.

33   Mckeown, T. (1990), 'The road to health', *World Health Forum*, vol. 10

34   World Bank (1993), *World Development Report.*

CHAPTER 2

Inequity in health

Inequities in health are defined as differences which are unnecessary and avoidable and judged to be unjust and unfair (Whitehead 1990: p. 6)[1]. Thus biological variations do not fall into this category and nor does health-damaging behaviour if it is freely chosen such as participation in certain sports and pastimes. What are clearly inequitable are restrictions of choice of lifestyle, exposure to unhealthy living and working conditions and inadequate access to essential health and other public services. Equity is, therefore, concerned with creating more equal opportunities for health and reducing differentials to the minimum.

Inequity in health can be looked at in a variety of ways. One of the most obvious is differences between geographical areas both within and between countries. A second is between different ethnic groups in the population, not only within developing countries but also in Europe as a result of the substantial immigration to Europe since the Second World War, particularly of persons from Asia, North Africa and the Caribbean. A third is differences between occupations which can be classified into social classes. A fourth is between those with jobs and those who are unemployed. A fifth is between those with different levels of educational achievement. A sixth is between income groups. Finally there are the differences between the sexes.

There are vast differences in health status between developed and developing countries. In Bangladesh, for example, one out of eight children die before they reach the age of one, while in Japan the figure is 1 in 142 and in Scandinavia 1 in 125. The death rate among children 1–4 years of age is around 20 per 1,000 in sub-Saharan Africa and in developed countries less than 1 per 1,000. Of the 20 million children born with low birth weight in 1985, 13 million were in South Asia and 3 million in Africa (WHO 1986: p. 26)[2]. The high death rate among the very young in developing countries results from diseases that have almost disappeared or been brought under control in developed countries. The main causes are the communicable diseases. These are often transmitted by human contact, insects, water, or inadequate sanitation. In developed countries, the elderly are the most vulnerable group with diseases of the circulatory system, cancers and the degenerative disorders of aging (WHO 1986: p. 20)[3].

Inequity in health in developing countries

A special problem of studying health inequalities in developing countries is the fact that in most of them the registration of births and deaths is seriously incomplete and, in some, a considerable proportion of the population cannot state their age with any accuracy. Local surveys can, however, be used to estimate infant mortality rates. Second, accurate data on income is difficult to collect as a high proportion of the working population works in the informal sector. But it is often possible to make comparisons between poorer and richer areas or between white and black populations. For example, it was found at independence (1980) in Zimbabwe that, in the capital (Harare), infant mortality was 14 per 1,000 among whites and between 30 and 50 per 1,000 among blacks; in the rural areas it was 140 to 200 per 1,000 for blacks (WHO 1987: p. 34)[4]. A UNICEF study of China[5] estimated that 41 cities and urban areas had infant mortality rates of less than 14 per thousand and 84 counties less than 24 per thousand. But there were over 500 counties with infant mortality rates over 50 per thousand live births, 265 counties with over 75 and 89 counties (not including Tibet) with over 100 per thousand. In South Africa, the African infant mortality was between 94 and 124 per 1,000 in 1981–85. The corresponding rates for Coloureds were 52, for Indians 18 and for Whites 12 (Centre of the Study of Health Policy 1988: p. 11)[6]. In rural Peru in the Andean provinces where the indigenous people live, the infant mortality rate is above 270 per 1,000, rising to 500 per 1,000 in isolated communities; in the wealthier districts of the capital it drops to 15 per 1,000 (WHO 1987: p. 41)[7]. In Indonesia, India and Kenya, child mortality is higher in states or provinces with larger proportions of poor people; within cities there are large differences in child mortality rates between rich and poor neighbourhoods (World Bank 1993: p. 40)[8].

In most developing countries, infants born in rural areas have a much lower chance of survival than urban infants. But in some, particularly in Latin America, 'people living in peri-urban slums have the poor health profile of deprived rural areas' (WHO 1987: p. 24)[9]. The most vulnerable are farmers with inadequate resources, landless agricultural labourers with limited employment opportunities, the illiterate and the urban poor living in slums and shanties.

One would expect inequalities to be greater in developing countries simply because there is greater inequality in the distribution of income. It has been estimated that in the average developing country the top 10 per cent of households receive 40 per cent of income and the bottom 40 per cent receive 10 per cent of income. In the United Kingdom, the top 10 per cent of the population receive 21 per cent of income and the bottom 50 per cent receive 25 per cent. Extreme poverty is very damaging to health particularly through malnutrition. Poor nourishment reduces resistance to disease, poor children do not absorb food so well and often it is wasted in debilitating diarrhoea and shared with invading parasites. Malnourishment in a child leads to both poor physical development and poor mental development. The underfed child is less able to absorb education.

Inequity in health in Europe

In Europe, inequalities are measured in many different ways – by occupation, income, education and social circumstances.

Inequalities between social groups show up in most countries when chronic disease and limiting long-standing illness are measured, with middle-aged men commonly showing rates of chronic disease 40 to 50 per cent higher in the lowest compared with the highest social groups. (Whitehead 1992: p. 291)[10]

In both Italy and Spain worse health in poorer groups, neighbourhoods and regions have been documented, with narrowing differences in post-neonatal mortality in Spain and widening differences in infant mortality in Italy between North and South (Whitehead 1992: p. 296)[11]. In France 2.8 times more mortality was found in adult men with low-grade jobs than in men with high-grade jobs with the gap widening between the late 1950s and the late 1970s (Whitehead 1992: p. 298)[12]. Socio-economic differentials have also been found in the Netherlands and they have widened since 1960.

The country in which health inequalities have been most intensively studied has been the United Kingdom. Data was brought together in the Black Report of 1980, updated in the Whitehead Report of 1987, and updated again in 1992. It is much easier to obtain data on occupation than income and then classify it into what are in effect social economic groupings. Early on in Britain a standard classification of occupations into social classes, taking into account skill and status, was developed for use in official statistics (see Table 2.1). The classification was originally devised for the census of population. But of critical importance for the present purpose is the fact that from 1911 onwards occupation has been required to be included on certificates of death and this social class classification has been used for mortality rates in conjunction with cause of death. The same social class classification is also frequently used in random surveys because of the convenience of comparison with census data. Thus differences in health by social class have been the focus of most work in Britain and the greatest controversies have focused around it.

There is some doubt whether the classification succeeds in accurately reflecting status or whose perceptions of status it reflects (see, e.g. Illsley and Le Grand 1987)[13]. But the classification does correlate fairly well with such factors as education and income. The intention is to group together people with broadly similar living

Table 2.1   **British system of occupational categories**

I	Professional (e.g. lawyer, doctor, accountant)
II	Intermediate (e.g. teacher, nurse, manager)
IIIa	Skilled non-manual (e.g. typist, shop assistant)
IIIb	Skilled manual (e.g. miner, bus driver, cook)
IV	Partly skilled manual (e.g. farm worker, bus conductor)
V	Unskilled manual (e.g. cleaner, labourer)

standards and ways of life. This was the justification for the uncomfortable sexist procedure of classifying married women by their husband's occupation, though they can now be classified by their own occupation.

In 1990 infant mortality rate for class V (the unskilled) was at least twice that of class I (professional) (Whitehead 1992: p. 230)[14]. In Denmark, however, differences between occupational groups in neonatal mortality have narrowed and were almost eliminated by 1977. This shows that such inequalities are not a natural law (Whitehead 1992: p. 301)[15]. Sweden has also managed to reduce the threefold differences between social groups in infant mortality found in the 1930s to about 10 per cent (Whitehead 1992: p. 306)[16].

Table 2.2   **Standardised mortality rate by cause 1979–83 (men aged 20–64)**

	Non-manual	Manual	Ratio
All causes	80	116	0.69
Lung cancer	65	129	0.50
Coronary health disease	87	114	0.76
Cerebro-vascular disease	76	120	0.63

Source: Whitehead (1992), p. 232.

Though the numbers are small, there are also differences in mortality rates in the United Kingdom by social class among persons of working age, with a greater difference for men than for women. The difference persists into old age but to a lesser extent. What however is important is that these differences are not just due to a few important diseases but are to be found in nearly all causes of death (see Table 2.2). It is even true of coronary heart disease, stroke and peptic ulcer – the confusingly named 'diseases of affluence'. These also cause a higher incidence of death in the poorer social classes than the richer. Indeed a study of the British Army in 1973–77 found that mortality from coronary heart disease was six times greater in the lowest than the highest ranks. Differences by type of housing, educational achievement and car ownership are shown in Table 2.3.

Table 2.3 **Standardised mortality rate (men aged 15+ in 1971)**

Housing	
Owner-occupied	84
Privately rented	109
Local authority	115
Education (aged 18–70)	
Degree	59
Other higher qualification	80
A levels only	91
Other	103
Access to car	
One or more	85
None	121

Source: Goldblatt, P. (1990), 'Mortality and alternative classifications', in Goldblatt, P. (ed.) *Longitudinal Study 1971–81: Mortality and Social Organisation*, OPCS, LS series, No. 6, HMSO, London.

Inequalities in mortality among working age adults are greater in France than in England and Wales, Hungary and Finland and smallest in Denmark, Norway and Sweden (Whitehead 1992: pp. 308–9)[17]. In Oslo, men in the two lowest socio-economic classes were two to three times more likely to die from cardiovascular disease than those in the professional classes. Particularly at risk were people whose jobs involved stress and monotony, and left little room for employees to influence the way their work was carried out. A study in Sweden found lung cancer highest among miners, insulation workers, type-setters and sheet-metal workers. In Finland, fatal accidents in men aged 35–64 were three times higher among unskilled blue-collar workers than among white-collar workers (WHO 1986: p. 43)[18].

Not only do the lower occupational groups have higher death rates but they experience more sickness and ill health throughout their lives. The unskilled manual group in the United Kingdom has twice the rate of limiting long-standing illness compared with the professional group. This is true for both men and women. It is not quite as marked for long-standing illness without limitation. In the case of acute sickness the difference does not occur until after age 45. The greatest differences in morbidity by social class are in the age group 45–64. The differences are shown between income groups in Table 2.4. Wide differences are also found between social classes in other dimensions of health such as perceived health, fitness and well-being. In the United States, compared with the highest fifth of income, those with the lowest fifth of income had more than twice as many days of restricted activity, more than twice as many days in bed due to illness, injury or impairment, and four times as many persons reported themselves to be in fair or poor health (Terris 1992: p. 35)[19]. Class gradients have been found in height, weight, birth weight, eye defects, and dental health in many countries (RUHBC 1989: p. 88)[20].

Table 2.4 **Percentage of income group suffering from morbidity**

	Poorest 20%	Richest 20%
Acute illness	24.6	18.5
Long-standing illness	24.3	17.1
Limited long-standing illness	28.8	13.9
Reporting 'not good health'	34.8	9.2

Source: O'Connell, O. and Propper, C. (1990), 'Equity and the distribution of National Health Service resources', *Journal of Health Economics*, vol. 10, no. 1, pp. 1–20.

Growing inequalities?

That all these differences exist is not disputed. What has caused controversy is whether they have become wider or narrower and why they exist. Comparisons over time are difficult to make for a number of reasons. First, there is the problem of data reliability: what is recorded on death certificates may be imprecise or inaccurate compared with what is ascertained at the Census. Second, occupations are reclassified into different social classes from time to time. Third, the relative proportions of the population in the different groups have been changing substantially over time. Membership of the highest two social classes has been expanding and that of the lowest contracting.

Of course it is true that nearly all health indicators improve for the population as a whole over time. What is in dispute is whether the relative decline is similar for the different social classes – whether relative inequalities have been expanding or contracting. From the figures available to it, the Black Report pointed out the extent to which relative inequalities among adults had been growing, particularly for men, over a period of 20 years; the picture for children was more variable (Townsend *et al.* 1982: pp. 6–7)[21]. The Whitehead

Table 2.5 **Trends in standardised mortality of men aged 25–64 by social class (Ratio from the average 1976–83)**

	1976–81	1981–83
Non-manual	84	83
Manual	103	107

Source: Whitehead (1992), p. 272.

Report pointed out, using a further decade of figures, that while there have been some improvements among children, the gap had been widening for adults (see Table 2.5).

A number of ways of checking on these findings have been used. Calculations have been made of how much difference the reclassification of occupations could have made. Findings from the more recent longitudinal study which links data sources have been analysed. Alternative classifications have been used such as the level of educational attainment, the Gini coefficient, the Slope Index of Inequality and the Index of Dissimilarity (Preston *et al.* 1981: pp. 233–54)[22]. They do not all suggest that inequalities in adults have been widening. But several comparisons have been taken back to the early 1930s and have argued that inequality has been growing over a period of 40 years.

Social classes are not evenly distributed over the United Kingdom. Thus it is not surprising to find regional differences in health indicators which have persisted, on average, for many years. Mortality rates are best towards the South and South East of Britain and tend to get worse as one goes north and particularly north-west of London or as one goes west or over the sea to Northern Ireland. Moreover the mortality gap between social classes widens as one goes north (see Table 2.6). But while age and sex standardised mortality show persistent differences over time, there has been a remarkable convergence in age-specific mortality rates among younger people but not among older age groups (Illersley and Le Grand (1994)[23]. Regional variations

Table 2.6 **Age-standardised mortality by region (Men aged 20–64)**

Region	Mortality per 1,000
Central Clydeside	7.9
Strathclyde	7.1
Rest of Scotland	6.1
Wales	5.9
York and Humberside	5.8
West Midlands	5.7
East Midlands	5.3
South East	4.9
South West	4.8
East Anglia	4.3
Britain	5.6

Source: Townsend, P. *et al.* (1984), *Inequalities in Health in the Northern Region*, NRHA, Bristol University.

are also to be found for data on disease and fitness and, at least within England, for rates of chronic disease. The variation is found for most disease conditions. More recent studies have broken down the data into smaller areas and it has been found that within high mortality regions there are communities which have as good mortality rates as anywhere in the world (GGHB 1984)[24]. These are, not surprisingly, the prosperous communities. Nevertheless, the high mortality regions have the greatest concentrations of material deprivation. A considerable amount of inter-regional and inter-area variations can be explained by occupational differences and levels of unemployment, but not all.

Health and unemployment

A considerable amount of work has been done relating unemployment to health. The unemployed have been shown to have higher mortality rates particularly from lung cancer, suicide, accidents and heart diseases (Moser *et al.* 1984: pp. 1324–28)[25]. One study in Edinburgh found an 11 to 1 difference in attempted suicide rates between the employed and the unemployed, with the incidence increasing neatly with the duration of unemployment (see Table 2.7). The unemployed also have more chronic sickness (Arber 1987: pp. 1069–73)[26]. And poorer health has been found in the children of the unemployed (Maclure and Stewart 1984: pp. 682–88)[27].

Table 2.7   Ratio of risk of attempted suicide between unemployed and employed (Edinburgh 1978–82)

Duration of unemployment	
Less than 6 months	6:1
6–12 months	10:1
Over 12 months	19:1

Source: Platt and Kreitman (1964), 'Unemployment and parasuicide in Edinburgh' *British Medical Journal*, 289, pp. 1029–32.

How far is the poor health of the unemployed explained by the fact that the incidence of unemployment is higher in the lower social classes? Are people with a high incidence of sickness more likely to lose their jobs? A longitudinal study followed men seeking work over a ten-year period and was able to control for occupation. It found 21 per cent of excess mortality (Moser *et al.* 1987: pp. 1324–28)[28]. This study focused on those actively seeking work and thus excludes the possibility that these men became unemployed because they already had poor health. What is interesting is that the wives of the 'seeking work' group also had excessive mortality, which may be due to low income. Another study followed up school leavers and found increasing psychiatric symptoms in those who became unemployed, and reduced symptoms in those who found work (Banks and Jackson 1982: pp. 789–98)[29]. Evidence is accumulating in Britain, as elsewhere, that unemployment can actually cause ill health.

The causes of inequalities

How can these inequalities be explained? It has already been shown that the hypotheses that they are due to poorly recorded data or problems of measurement over time must be discarded. Are they due to failings in the health service? At first sight this might seem impossible in Britain, which has a national health service readily available to all citizens with only some relatively small charges. But the story is not as simple as that. While everybody can use the health service, access is not as easy for all social groups. For example, one study has shown that doctors tend to be concentrated in the better off rather than the deprived areas of a town and people with a car clearly found it easier to get to a doctor (Knox 1979: pp. 160–68)[30]. Dental services also tend to be concentrated in better-off districts (Carmichael 1985: pp. 24–27)[31]. There is evidence that the lower social classes are less likely to use preventive, ophthalmic, dental and chiropody services (Richie *et al.* 1981)[32]. One study found that higher social class patients received more explanations of their health problems than lower class patients (Penleton and Bochner 1980: pp. 669–73)[33] and another showed that the higher social classes were more likely to receive home visits (Bucquet *et al.* 1985: pp. 1480–83)[34]. The higher social classes are also more likely to be referred to specialists than lower class patients (Blaxter 1984: pp. 1963–67)[35]. And for any given sickness, the higher social classes are more likely to go to a doctor (OPCS 1982–1990)[36]. While these studies have shown that the health service does not actually succeed in providing equal access for equal need as intended, these failings can probably only be implicated to a marginal extent in an attempt to explain health inequalities.

One hypothesis which has been put forward is a Darwinian theory of natural selection. People with poor health move down the social scale and people with good health move up the social scale. Studies have shown, for example, that shorter women tend to move down the social scale on marriage and the taller move up (Knight 1984)[37]. It has also been found that boys who have had serious illnesses tend to fall down the social scale by the age of 26 (Wadsworth 1988: pp. 50–74)[38]. But it has been shown that the numbers involved in these inter-class movements are far too small to have much effect on the total figures (Wilkinson 1986: pp. 151–66)[39]. Moreover a study has shown no effect of this kind for older adults (Fox *et al.* 1988)[40].

Thus there remain explanations of health inequalities in terms of behaviour and explanations in terms of material circumstances, though they are closely associated. Some put all the blame on the lower social classes for causing their own poor health. They quote the extensive evidence of differences in behaviour between the social classes. While in 1972 the proportion of men in the highest social class who smoked cigarettes was 33 per cent, by 1984 the proportion had dropped to 17 per cent. The lowest social class had much higher rates in both years and much less of a fall. The figures for men were 64 per cent for 1972 and still 49 per cent for 1984. In 1984, heavy drinkers of alcohol were 26 per cent of men in the lowest social class and 8 per cent in the highest social class (Whitehead 1992: pp. 290–93)[41]. In the late 1970s the lower income groups ate more white bread, sugar, fats and potatoes than the higher income groups, but by the late 1980s many of the differences had almost disappeared (Whitehead 1992: p. 293)[42]. The higher social classes take a great deal more exercise than the lowest social class, and so on.

Three important points must be made about this controversy. First, it is unrealistic to draw a hard and fast line between behaviour and material factors, as material circumstances are in part responsible for behaviour. For example, a healthy diet is more expensive than an unhealthy diet. Smoking and heavy drinking are ways of coping with stress, and giving children sweets is an easy way of keeping them quiet on a shopping trip.

Second, if behaviour or lifestyle were wholly responsible for health inequalities, one would expect to find the differences in mortality between social classes wholly due to diseases associated with these lifestyles. But this is not the case. For all the major causes of death there are social class differences in mortality rates.

Third, social class variations have been controlled for risk factors. A study of civil servants found, in the case of mortality from coronary heart disease, that controlling for age, smoking, and blood pressure, height and blood sugar explained under 25 per cent of the social class differences in mortality (Marmot *et al.* 1984: pp. 1003–6)[43]. In the case of the unemployed, controlling for smoking and alcohol consumption did not remove the excess mortality (Cook *et al.* 1982: pp. 1290–94)[44]. A study in Alameda County in California examined the risk of death over an eighteen-year period where the poor had over twice the mortality rate. After controlling for 13 factors including smoking, exercise and race, it found that the risk of death was still one and a half times greater for the poor (Kaplan 1985)[45].

Once again, evidence is accumulating on how bad housing or cheap housing can harm health with high rates of infectious diseases, respiratory disease and mental illness (DoE 1981)[46]. Poorly designed buildings can also cause serious accidents in children (DoE 1981)[47]. And families who are economizing on fuel risk making their homes cold, damp and prone to condensation. The level of pollution is also important.

Working conditions are also significant and not only in the context of accidents. Factory workers are exposed to chemicals, noise and dust which can lead to a variety of disorders. Not only are they exposed to hazardous substances, but they may take contaminants home on their clothing and skin. It has also been calculated that lung cancer and emphysema are related to working conditions, even when smoking is controlled for (RUHBC 1989: p. 105)[48].

Income is still an important variable. A study has shown that in the period 1951 to 1971 occupations with a relative increase in earnings tended to experience a relative decrease in mortality rates and vice versa (Wilkinson 1988: pp. 88–114)[49]. While there has been virtually no correlation between increases in gross national product per head and increases in life expectancy in the OECD countries, there is a strong correlation between income distribution and life expectancy. Countries with a more equal income distribution had higher life expectancy. Moreover, among the European Community countries falls in relative poverty have been significantly related to a faster improvement in life expectancy (Whitehead 1992: p. 330)[50]. Over the past 30 years life expectancy has improved in Western Europe, but deteriorated in Central and Eastern Europe. This was associated with the fall in living standards of the latter (Dahlgren and Whitehead 1992: p. 3)[51]. All the ways in which income, directly or indirectly, influences health are not known and this is clearly an area where more research is needed. But, with present knowledge, material circumstances seem to be more important than lifestyle even though we do not know in depth precisely why.

The health of minority ethnic groups

What evidence is there about the health of minority ethnic groups? The mortality rates for most immigrant groups have been lower than those in their countries of birth. The exception is in the case of immigrants from Ireland (Marmot *et al.* 1984)[52]. All immigrant groups have higher mortality than the average for England and Wales for tuberculosis and accidents but lower in the case of bronchitis. Immigrants from the Indian sub-continent have low mortality for several cancers common in the United Kingdom, but higher mortality from liver cancer, heart disease and diabetes. Infant mortality rates are strikingly high for mothers born in Pakistan and quite high for mothers born in the Caribbean. Puzzlingly, people of Asian origin have high rates of coronary heart disease despite a low prevalence of smoking and low consumption of alcohol. Are the high rates due to poverty, the stress of immigration or discrimination? The question is still unanswered.

Sex differences

Sex differences are particularly interesting. Why was it that by 1983 a girl in the United Kingdom could expect to live six years longer than a boy – an improvement of two whole years since 1971 – an extraordinarily rapid improvement? In developed countries the expectation of life of females is between five and ten times longer than that of men. Why is it that males die more often than females in every age group from birth through adulthood yet women consistently record higher levels of chronic and acute sickness. Why are most psychiatric problems found in married women? Paid employment seems to reduce illness in middle-class women but increase it in working-class women (Cox *et al.* 1987)[53].

The obvious explanation for male/female differences is genetic. But environment can clearly be very important. In India and Papua New Guinea, men live longer than women. Part of the reason is high maternal mortality. One study has estimated that half the difference in survival rates in the United Kingdom can be explained by behaviour such as cigarette smoking, alcohol consumption and occupational hazards (Waldron 1987: pp. 349–62)[54]. A study has shown that in Kibbutz life in Israel, where there is less difference in gender roles and a similar environment, the male/female gap in life expectancy is about half what would be expected due to higher male life expectancy (Leviathan and Cohen 1985: pp. 545–51)[55].

Conclusion

Damaging health behaviours are social class correlated but those that are known seem to explain much less than half of the social class variations, and some lifestyles are strongly influenced by the social environment. On the other hand, evidence of the importance of materialist (or structural) factors has been growing. The case for greater equality has long been argued for a variety of reasons – solidarity, social cohesion or just plain justice. But it is now recognised increasingly that excess inequality is not just unfair but is in addition health-damaging. Societies which have less inequality in income, less variations in housing standards and better working conditions seem to have less health inequalities between socio-economic groups.

Notes

1   Whitehead, M. (1990), *The Concepts and Principles of Equity and Health*, WHO, Copenhagen.
2   World Health Organisation (1986), *Intersectoral Action for Health*, WHO, Geneva.

3   WHO (1986), *Intersectoral Action*.
4   World Health Organisation (1987), *Financing Health Development*, WHO (HSC) Geneva.
5   Quoted in World Bank (1991), *China: Long-term Issues and Options in the Health Transition*, vol. 1, p. 7, World Bank, Washington, D.C.
6   Centre of the Study of Health Policy (1985), *A National Health Service for South Africa: The Case for Change*, Witwatersrand University, Johannesburg.
7   WHO (1987), *Financing Health Development*.
8   World Bank (1993), *World Development Report 1993: Issues in Health*, World Bank, Washington D.C.
9   WHO (1987), *Financing Health Development*.
10 Whitehead, M. (1992), *The Health Divide*, Penguin, Harmondsworth.
11 Whitehead (1992), *The Health Divide*.
12 Whitehead (1992), *The Health Divide*.
13 Illersley, R. and Le Grand, J. (1987), 'The measurement of inequality in health', in Williams, A. (ed.), *Economics and Health*, London.
14 Whitehead (1992), *The Health Divide*.
15 Whitehead (1992), *The Health Divide*.
16 Whitehead (1992), *The Health Divide*.
17 Whitehead (1992), *The Health Divide*.
18 WHO (1986), *Intersectoral Action*.
19 Terris, M. (1992), 'Budget cutting and privatization: the threat to health', *Journal of Public Health Policy*, vol. 13, no. 1.
20 Research Unit in Health and Behavioural Change (RUHBC) (1989), *Changing the Public Health*, Wiley, Chichester.
21 Townsend, P. *et al.* (1982), *The Black Report*, Penguin, Harmondsworth.
22 Preston, S. *et al.* (1981), 'Effects of industrialisation on mortality in developed countries', *Solicited Papers*, vol. 2, IUSSP, Manila.
23 Illersley R. and Le Grand, J. (1994), 'Regional inequalities in mortality', *Journal of Epidemiology and Community Health*.
24 Greater Glasgow Health Board (1984), *Ten Year Report 1974–83)*, GGHB, Glasgow.
25 Moser, K.A. *et al.* (1984), 'Unemployment and mortality in the OPCS Longitudinal Study', *Lancet*, vol. ii.
26 Arber, S. (1987), 'Social class, non-employment and chronic illness', *British Medical Journal*, vol. 294.
27 Maclure, A. and Stewart, G.T. (1984), 'Admission of children to hospital in Glasgow: relation to unemployment and other deprivation variables', *Lancet*, vol. ii.
28 Moser, K.A. *et al.* (1987), 'Unemployment and Mortality'.
29 Banks, M.H. and Jackson, P.R. (1982), 'Unemployment and the risk of minor psychiatric disorder in young people', *Psychological Medicine*, vol. 123.
30 Knox, P.L. (1979), 'The accessibility of primary care to urban patients: a geographical analysis', *Journal of the Royal College of General Practitioners*, vol. 29 (220).
31 Carmichael, C.L. (1985), 'Inner city Britain: a challenge for the dental profession', *British Dental Journal*, vol. 159, no. 1.
32 Richie, J. *et al.* (1981), *Access to Primary Health Care*, OPCS, HMSO, London.
33 Penleton, D.A. and Bochner, A. (1980), 'The communication of medical

information in general practice as a function of patients' social class', *Social Science and Medicine*, vol. 14.

34   Bucquet, D. *et al.* (1985), 'Factors associated with home visiting in an inner London general practice', *British Medical Journal*, vol. 290.

35   Blaxter, M. (1984), 'Equality and consultation rates in general practice', *British Medical Journal*, vol. 288.

36   OPCS (1982–1990), *General Household Surveys*, OPCS, HMSO, London.

37   Knight, I. (1984), *The Height and Weight of Adults in Great Britain*, OPCS, HMSO, London.

38   Wadsworth, M.E.J. (1988), 'Serious illness in childhood and its association with later life achievement', in Wilkinson, R.J. (ed.), *Class and Health, Research and Longitudinal Data*, Tavistock, London.

39   Wilkinson, R.G. (1986), 'Occupational class, selection and inequalities in health', *Quarterly Journal of Social Affairs*, vol. 2, no. 4.

40   Fox, A.J. *et al.* (1988), 'Social class mobility differentials: artefact of life circumstances?' in Wilkinson, R.G. (ed.), *Class and Health*.

41   Whitehead (1992), *The Health Divide*.

42   Whitehead (1992), *The Health Divide*.

43   Marmot, M.G. *et al.* (1984), 'Inequalities in death specific explanations of a general pattern', *Lancet*, vol. ii.

44   Cook, D.G. *et al.* (1982), 'Health of unemployed middle-aged men in Great Britain', *Lancet*, vol. i.

45   Kaplan, G.A. (1985), 'Twenty years of Health in Alameda County: the Human Laboratory Analyses', paper presented at the Society for Prospective Medicine, Annual Meeting, San Francisco, 24 November 1985.

46   Department of the Environment (1981), *An Investigation of Difficult to Let Housing*, HMSO, London

47   Department of the Environment (1981), *People in Flats*, HMSO, London.

48   RUHBC (1989), *Changing the Public Health*.

49   Wilkinson, R.G. (1988), 'Income and mortality' in Wilkinson *Class and Health*.

50   Whitehead (1992), *The Health Divide*.

51   Dahlgren. G. and Whitehead, M. (1992), *Policies and Strategies to Promote Equity in Health*, WHO, Copenhagen.

52   Marmot, M.G. *et al.* (1984), 'Immigrant mortality in England and Wales 1970–78', in OPCS, *Studies of Medical and Population Subjects*, no. 47, HMSO, London.

53   Cox, B. *et al.* (1987), 'Health and life style survey', Health Promotion Trust, London.

54   Waldron, I. (1987), 'Why do women live longer than men?', *Social Science and Medicine*, vol. 24.

55   Leviathan, U. and Cohen, J. (1985), 'Gender differences in life expectancy among kibbutz members', *Social Science and Medicine*, vol. 21.

CHAPTER 3

Lifestyle and health promotion

Lifestyle is defined as the way of life which, in theory, is within the choice of the individual, however limited the range of choice may be. At first sight, changing lifestyles might seem to be the easiest and cheapest way of securing health improvement in a society at any level of development. If people in developing countries learned to boil their water, bury their faeces and household waste and select or grow the most nutritious diet which is within their means, health status would show a notable improvement. Similarly if people in both developed and developing countries did not smoke, take alcohol in excess, were safety conscious on the roads and at work, a large amount of morbidity and mortality could be avoided.

Knowledge is not enough

At first sight it may seem that all that is needed is to give people health knowledge and they are bound to respond to it, because everyone sees the importance of health. But life is far from being that simple. To a large extent people are prisoners of their values and the values of the society they live in, and are limited by their economic and social environment quite apart from any health knowledge they may possess. Thus it is no use blaming the victims of unhealthy behaviours. An authoritarian society may be able to some extent to impose health on people whether they like it or not. But in most societies this would be unacceptable, except in very limited contexts. Thus it is necessary to understand the different and often conflicting pressures to which different groups of people are subject. Without this understanding, attempts to change health behaviours may not just be ineffective but counterproductive.

In some societies, values, beliefs and social and economic pressures may coincide. The predominant value might be fatalism. There is nothing you can do to alter your future which is pre-ordained. Ill health must be accepted as the punishment of the gods or as evil spirits planted by others. This belief comes from the elders and the religious teachers. And it is reinforced by all the pressures of the social environment, both kinship and community. In some societies, fatalism may be no more than a response to the hopelessness people feel about ever changing the circumstances of their life in which they see themselves as permanently locked.

In some other societies, the relationships are much more complicated. Most societies, even 'developed' have a lay view of health which does not correspond completely with the Cartesian scientific pluralism which underlies allopathic medicine (RUHBC 1989: p. 32)[1]. The allopathic doctor looks for an efficient treatment of the physical cause of symptoms and tends to exclude any serious interest in the complexity of the life situation in which the patient is immersed. 'Traditional' practitioners broadly divide into two groups (Foster 1983: p. 19)[2]. There are those who see symptoms as caused by the purposeful intervention of sensate agents (deities, evil spirits, or sorcerers) who seek out a victim who falls ill. Aggression or punishment is directed against a single person as a consequence of the will and power of a human or supernatural agent. Others see symptoms as caused by an upset in body humours and consequent loss of bodily equilibrium. The intrusions of hot or cold into the body or their loss upsets its equilibrium which must be restored if the patient is to recover. The first group predominates in the traditional systems of Africa, Oceania and indigenous Siberia though naturalistic explanations may be present as well. They also underlie the more complex systems of contemporary China, South Asia and Latin America. The second group predominates in Ayurvedic, Urani and traditional Chinese medicine.

These beliefs may be shared by the patient in whole or part. This is why people often accept the services of allopathic doctors and also use traditional rituals and ceremonies (Foster 1983: p. 21)[3]. The allopathic doctor alleviates the symptoms but until the ultimate cause is uncovered and dealt with, improvement will be temporary. Even people with a scientific education may still act in this way, showing a conflict between the values of the traditional society and the beliefs learnt through education. For those with deep roots in the traditional way of thinking, it is difficult to expect them to accept, for example, that clean water, mosquitoes, flies and snails are relevant to health. It was first assumed in Chiapas (Mexico) that respected traditional healers would be the best intermediaries for promoting socio-cultural change. It was later found that health training for young literate people was a more practical approach to providing primary health care (Foster 1983: p. 23)[4].

Allopathic medicine is sometimes called 'scientific' medicine but not all of it justifies this term, in so far as by no means all allopathic treatments have been verified by random controlled trials. Other systems of medicine have been found to get better results for certain conditions, but the extent that this is so is not known as nearly all scientific effort at verifying the results of treatment have been done on allopathic medicine and not on the other, often much older, systems of treatment.

Preventive medicine plays a part in traditional medicine. In Latin America cold air must be avoided. In Africa, preventive practices include immunisations; the wearing of conservation objects to stave off illnesses; sacrifices and offerings; and the observance of prohibitions, taboos and a number of rituals of bodily hygiene (Koumare 1983: p. 27)[5]. In many traditional societies, houses and their surroundings must be meticulously cleaned and refuse burned or removed from the immediate vicinity of the house. Defecation often occurs in the fields or the surrounding bush. Further preventive messages can readily be built on this last basis by showing how flies can bring it back into the house or how it can infect children with hookworm.

What is important is that, wherever possible, the message does not defy the values of the society. In societies where an imbalance of 'hot' and 'cold' foods are thought to cause illness, nutrition messages need to be adapted to these beliefs. For example, menstruation is thought to be a 'warm' state, so 'cold' foods should be avoided because they might cause cramps. As pregnancy is also a 'warm' state foods defined as 'cold' must be avoided (RUHBC 1989: p. 33)[6]. It was found that Puerto Rican women avoided vitamins and iron because these were considered 'hot' (Harwood 1971: pp. 1153–68)[7]. In societies where women should be isolated during lactation, it is easier to promote longer lactation and therefore greater birth spacing than the use of contraceptives. Where, as in Ghana, sex is the primary reason for a friendship between a man and a woman, 'any AIDS educational effort that attempts to suggest alternatives to penetrative sex is likely to fail' (Ankomah 1922: p. 139)[8]. It was found in Peru that:

to understand fully the varieties of response to the water boiling issue, it was necessary to take into account many sectors of culture, including definitions of health and illness, the organisation of kitchens and the scheduling of daily chores, mobility aspirations, the prevailing status system, and community's patterns of utilisation of water resources. (Wellin 1982: pp. 16–18)[9].

It takes great courage for a mother to break with tradition whether in boiling water when well or breaking a food taboo. Health cannot be imposed on people. It has to be won in partnership with them.

In developed countries, there may also be a conflict between values and knowledge. The value is still fatalistic: life chances depend on luck – what job you get or whether you win the football pools. It is your luck whether smoking and drinking damages your health, and to some extent this is true. There is no point in planning for the future. Taking risks is showing manly courage. For example, it is sexy to drive a motor cycle as fast as it will go. On the other hand it may be accepted as knowledge that smoking can damage your health. Only about 4 per cent of British people deny that smoking is bad for your health and only 7 per cent deny that alcohol is bad for your health. But much higher proportions of the population smoke and drink. Changing knowledge does not necessarily change behaviour (RUHBC 1989: p. 70)[10].

The deciding influences on behaviour are often social pressures – what the peer group does. Social life may be built around the pub where nearly everyone smokes, and offering a cigarette may be a standard chatting-up approach. These behaviours may be reinforced by what celebrities are said to do or are portrayed as doing in the advertisements. Social pressures are often strong enough to resist economic pressures. It costs money to smoke and drink but it is a price that has to be paid to participate in social life. Or economic pressures may reinforce social pressures. Healthy foods, at least in Britain, are not only more expensive than unhealthy foods (see Table 3.1.), but they also take longer to prepare. For those in low income groups, time as well as money costs can be important determinants of behaviour.

Table 3.1   **The cost of a recommended diet**

NOT RECOMMENDED	Pence	RECOMMENDED	Pence
White bread	3.4	Wholemeal bread	4.7
Whole milk	9.3	Skimmed milk	18.4
Cheddar cheese	8.1	Reduced fat cheese	18.8
Mince	17.7	Lean beef	33.0
Fatty pork	11.3	Lean pork	42.6
Sausages	9.4	Poultry	34.7
Canned fruit	18.0	Fresh fruit	30.8

Source: Lang, T. *et al.* (1986), *Tightening Belts,* London Food Commission, London.

Most people are highly responsive to social pressures, but not all. Psychologists make a distinction between outer-directed persons who are responsive to social pressures and inner directed persons – those who do their own thing and do not care what others do or what they think. Being outer-directed does not necessarily imply any greater health consciousness.

The value of planning for the future is to be found more with those with better education. The whole educational process of climbing the ladder by passing a series of examinations requires a willingness to sacrifice the present for the future. Not all are willing to do this. Having a job and earning one's own bread is seen as adult status and some grasp it as early as they can, even if there is not all that much bread and the amount is unlikely to increase much throughout life. A job, however insecure, is seen as better than continuing as a student with the dependency on parents that this implies. If people have never absorbed middle class aspiring values, it is useless to direct health education messages at them as if they had. If life is a matter of luck and the future can take care of itself, it is of little interest to be told what activities which give pleasure today run risks of major health damage in the future. To tell children of eleven that they may not live as long as their grandparents if they adopt some health-damaging behaviour may make no impact if the last thing that they want is to live long enough to suffer the afflictions of old age as they see them.

The better educated are better served by the media. It has been found that the 'quality' press publishes more articles on health; is more informative by citing books, articles and government reports; and gives more coverage of social factors in ill-health such as unemployment and class inequalities. A much higher proportion of articles are also published about prevention and health maintenance (RUHBC 1989: pp. 55–56)[11]. At its worst, the media can give false impressions. It was found in the case of the use of heroin that the media tended to reinforce the idea that a 'pusher' was an evil stranger, that heroin led to enslavement, that coming off was always very painful, and that the drug is instantly addictive – none of which is true (Pearson *et al.* 1985)[12].

This does not mean that attempts to change behaviour are bound to be fruitless – at least with some social groups who have value systems which do not resist change. Values, beliefs and social pressures can and do change over time, though the process by which they do may not be readily understood. Social pressures are certainly changing in Europe as well as in the United States. Smokers now usually have to ask permission to smoke, as was not the case 30 years ago. Indeed in some public situations, they are already beginning to feel like an oppressed minority. The trends in smoking behaviour in Britain are shown in Table 3.2.

Table 3.2 **Trends in cigarette smoking by sex and social class (1972 – 88)**

	I	II	IIIa	IIIb	IV	V	ALL
			Percentage smoking				
MEN							
1972	33	44	45	57	57	64	52
1978	25	37	38	49	53	60	45
1984	17	29	30	42	47	49	38
1988	16	26	25	39	40	43	30
WOMEN							
1972	33	38	38	47	42	42	42
1978	23	33	33	42	41	41	37
1984	15	29	28	37	37	36	32
1988	17	26	27	35	37	39	30

Source: OPCS, *General Household Surveys*, HMSO, London.

Smoking fell for both sexes and all social classes between 1972 and 1988. But the reduction in the lowest social class has been much lower than in the highest social class so that the gap between the social classes has widened. Women in the lowest social class smoked considerably less than men in 1972. But the reduction among women of the lowest social class has been less than among men so that by 1988 the rate of smoking among women was the same as for men. Between 1984 and 1988, the proportion of women smoking actually increased. Women responded to the special appeal made by the advertisers, particularly by suggesting subtly that smoking makes one thin and stressing the point by marketing slim cigarettes aimed at women (Amos 1990: pp. 416–38)[13]. In developing countries, smoking rates are increasing in both men and women ('Round table' 1990: pp. 3–13)[14]. The smoking habits of parents influence their children: mothers who smoke are likely to have children who smoke ('Round table' 1990: p. 10)[15].

While smoking has been on the decline in Europe and North America, the producers have been compensating for declining markets by putting their major efforts elsewhere. The target for the 1960s was Latin America. A British-owned firm now claims 80 per cent of the market in Brazil. In the 1970s and 1980s the target became Africa, the Middle East and the Far East: threats of trade sanctions prised open the markets of Taiwan, Korea and Japan and forced the latter to begin television advertising, though banned in the United States, until it leapt to second place in time allotments (Macalister 1992)[16]. From the late 1980s, the target was the opening market of Eastern Europe with the final target China. This market, which had been closed on ideological grounds, was estimated to have 40 per cent of world smokers (Macalister 1992)[17].

On the other hand, the consumption of alcohol continues to rise in most of Europe: the British figures are shown in Figure 3.1. The rise has been largely caused by the declining cost of alcohol in relation to real incomes with a switch from beer, which has become relatively more expensive, to wine and spirits (Maynard 1986: pp. 61–71)[18]. However, the campaign in Britain against drinking and driving has been a considerable success. Deaths and serious injuries from alcohol-related road accidents more than halved between 1979 and 1991. During the same period breath tests multiplied by three and the proportion of positive results fell from 42 per cent to 16 per cent (*Acquire* 1991: p. 2)[19]. A WHO study for some 50 countries found consumption increasing in both North and South America, though declining in most African countries and to a lesser extent in Asia, Oceania and in some countries of Europe (Smart 1991: pp. 99–103)[20].

The consumption of white bread is giving way to brown, and in this respect the lower social classes have largely caught up with the higher and there is now little difference in the social class variation in the consumption of animal fats. One of the large supermarket chains is

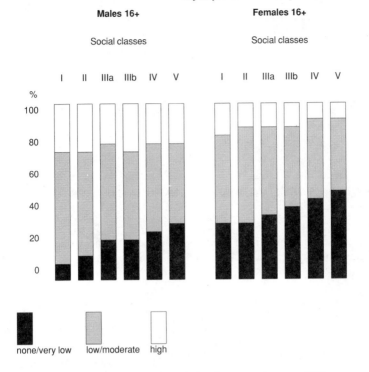

Males 16+

Females 16+

Social classes

Social classes

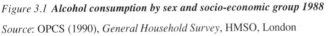

none/very low   low/moderate   high

*Figure 3.1 **Alcohol consumption by sex and socio-economic group 1988***

Source: OPCS (1990), *General Household Survey*, HMSO, London

researching on fatless bacon and, for the longer-term future, 'pigless bacon'. The range of fresh fruit has extended with imports from all over the world to defeat the seasons. Healthy foods are now clearly marked and often grouped together to try and win back the custom which has deserted them for health shops.

The trends in exercise are shown in Table 3.3. The steep variation by social class remains in 1986 as in 1977 with little change in the extent to which people walk over two miles. Swimming has become more popular in all social classes with the change much more concentrated in the higher social classes. Department stores have reacted to the craze for jogging and devote whole departments to sports shoes and custom track suits – some of which are never used for jogging.

In some ways economic progress has eased the task of being healthy. Europeans expect constant hot water and there are now few hotels which do not provide bathrooms and toilets *en suite*. The strenuous weekly wash and economy with clean laundry have gone out. The washing machine has replaced it, with one to every household in richer areas, and launderettes in poorer areas. The mass sales are of

Table 3.3   **Trends in exercise by social class (1977 and 1986)**

Social class	Walking over 2 miles		Indoor swimming	
	1977	1986	1977	1986
Ia	29	30	6	16
Ib	23	24	6	11
II	27	⎫	7	⎫
IIIa	20	⎬ 22	5	⎬ 12
IIIb	15	17	4	7
IV	12	15	1	7
V	10	12	2	3

Source: OPCS *General Household Surveys*, HMSO, London.

clothes which do not need ironing, leaving only higher priced prestige items which do.

The role of health promotion

Those whose task it is to try to get a message across have much to learn from the advertising industry, which has highly developed skills. And these skills can be used to promote health as well as to damage it. The rapid acceptance of toothpaste containing fluoride, which has done so much to reduce dental decay and the need for dentists, was due to the skills of advertisers, even though many professors of dentistry at first doubted its effectiveness. Advertisers have learnt from experience that it is no use producing a product unless it is known in advance who wants to buy it. The first step is to find out which groups in society by income group, sex, age and geographical area will want to buy and for what reason. Thus advertisers concentrate their efforts on reminding people what they know already and placing their product within this set of beliefs or wants. The character of the advertising is directed at the particular group where it is known the market is to be found. Thus the advertiser associates a product with masculinity, risk-taking and aggressiveness by using truck drivers, horse riders and pylon repairers. Or beer aimed at a working class clientele is associated with football players, boxers and the pub in advertisements where celebrities can be introduced. Expensive perfumes are associated with film stars dressed in silk and furs. Expensive cars are associated with expensive night clubs and restaurants. An advertisement shows by the images used what sex and income group it is aiming to reach.

Many past attempts at health education have defied these rules. They have dashed in blindly and aggressively without research to establish what the acceptance is likely to be or where the market is.

They have tried to use advertising to challenge deep-seated values and beliefs. The attempt to associate cigarette smoking with death and funerals was noticeably ineffective in the long term. Any change induced by fear tends to be short-lived (Whitehead 1989: p. 25)[21]. The immediate reaction from most of the audience is resistance or denial (RUHBC 1989: pp. 81–82)[22]. With young people it can have a reverse effect if it glamorises rare or novel behaviours; anything dangerous appeals to teenagers. Using fear directly is dangerous unless perhaps it is done with a light touch:

AIDS KILLS
DON'T BE SILLY
PUT A CONDOM
ON YOUR WILLY.

Telling regular smokers and drinkers not to smoke or drink is bound to be counterproductive (Whitehead 1989: p. 25)[23]. A positive message is always more effective than a negative image. Telling people how to give up smoking and testimonies from those who have succeeded in doing so are likely to make more impact than telling people what not to do. Not smoking can be associated with sexual attractiveness (and, indirectly, sexual achievement), sporting achievement, skin condition and other matters of profound interest to the young. Moreover the message may be put across more effectively by making an aesthetic appeal rather than a health appeal:

KISS A NON-SMOKER
AND TASTE THE DIFFERENCE,

or more crudely:

IF YOU PROMISE NOT TO SMOKE,
I WILL PROMISE NOT TO FART,

or

HE WAS OF NO USE TO ME
HE HAD DRUNK FAR TOO MUCH.

Margaret Whitehead sums up on substance abuse: 'Most of the ineffectual methods have one thing in common: they have tended to concentrate on the substance abused rather than the problems of the person or the social context in which abuses take place' (Whitehead 1989, p. 17)[24].

Those engaged in health promotion through the mass media or 'social marketing' need to apply similar methods to the advertisers: they need to know their market and try out slogans on target groups.

An alternative use of the mass media is 'media advocacy', stimulating media coverage of the ethical and legal culpability of the industries promoting unhealthy products – the 'merchants of death' trying to exploit children and putting profits before health and safety (Wallack 1990: pp. 150–52)[25].

In so far as skilled health promotion campaigns can gradually change behaviour, their impact is likely to be greater on the higher income groups than the lower. This is partly because the higher income groups have longer time horizons, and partly because better educated people are in a stronger position to analyse complex and conflicting messages coming from advertisers and health educators. This type of health promotion is likely to widen health inequalities. This does not mean that it should not be done but it does mean that special effort should be made to concentrate other types of campaigns on the lower income groups.

It has been learnt over the past ten years that face-to-face contact between health professionals and the public is one effective way of changing behaviour. General practitioners who offered patients who smoked advice on stopping, gave them a leaflet and warned that they would be followed up, achieved a 5.1 per cent cessation rate after one year, compared to 0.3 per cent for controls who were only asked if they smoked or not (Wallack 1990: p. 31)[26]. Nurses can be even more effective: in one study 17 per cent of the experimental group had given up smoking after a year following nurse counselling compared with 8.3 per cent of controls who had no counselling (Macleod-Clark *et al.* 1987)[27]. Attempts at health promotion are likely to be most successful when the economic and social environment is being changed at the same time, for example, by higher taxes of cigarettes and alcohol as discussed in the next chapter.

As pointed out earlier, giving people knowledge about what is favourable or unfavourable to health is far from being enough to influence health behaviour. And telling people what they should do is likely to be ineffective or even counter-productive. A much wider and more democratic approach is needed – health promotion. This has been defined by the World Health Organisation as 'the process of enabling people to increase control over and to improve their health' (WHO 1984)[28]. As one American critic points out, seeing lifestyles as

a social pattern and expression of culture, as the modus operandi of social life, as both a consequence of social structure and a mediating resource (a social buffer) has *not been* of great interest to public health interventionists. This has resulted in public health approaches which are, in my view, politically naive, hampered by a simple cause-effect mentality; often redundant of already established lay initiatives; stuck on clinical-experimental designs; often medicalising and rarely empowering; frequently stridently healistic; innocent of structural factors; and sometimes (at least in America) self-serving the desire of shrinking sick care institutions to capture 'new markets' for survival purposes (Levin 1982)[29].

Above all else, any attempt to improve lifestyles 'must be based on the choices that people in difficult circumstances can make, so that realistic, credible advice and help can be given' (Dahlgren and Whitehead 1992: p. 34)[30].

Health education in schools

A vital age group for health promotion is children aged 8 to 13. Experimenting with smoking can start as early as age nine and experimenting with glue and alcohol not long afterwards. The cause may be no more than the desire to enjoy illicitly what appear to be adult pleasures, forbidden to children. Experience has shown that health education should be comprehensive and not deal with isolated problems; it should be continued over the years with a substantial time commitment and the same themes should be repeated at different stages of the course. The training of the teachers is critical and the involvement of parents highly desirable. The aim is to help children clarify their ideas, values and attitudes (Whitehead 1989: p. 12)[31]. There is clear evidence in Britain that it can be effective in smoking ('my body project'), dental health ('natural gnashers'), exercise ('the Linwood project') and reducing teenage pregnancy (Whitehead 1989: p. 15)[32]. The more widespread sex education in the United Kingdom compared with the United States, coupled with reasonable access to contraceptive advice, have been key factors in keeping pregnancy rates lower in the United Kingdom (Jones *et al.* 1985: pp. 53–63)[33]. A clear failure has been with drug education in the United States: the methods aimed specifically at preventing drug abuse have been at best ineffective and at worst counter-productive (Jones *et al.* 1985: p. 16)[34].

Advertising

Attempts at health promotion have large barriers to overcome. The resources devoted to health education, in most countries, both developed and developing, are tiny, while the resources at the command of the advertisers of products which can be health-damaging are immense. The tobacco industry spends at least £100 million on advertising in the United Kingdom (King's Fund: p. 79)[35] and the alcohol industry £200 million (Whitehead 1989: p. 23)[36]. In the United States the tobacco industry spends US$ 2 billion on advertising and the average adolescent sees over 5,000 beer commercials in a year (Wallack 1990: p. 146–47)[37]: children can name more brands of beer than presidents of America (Wallack 1990: p. 152)[38]. And when magazines become heavily dependent on advertisements of particular types of product, this inevitably restrains editors from making strong criticism of them.

Compared to all this, expenditure on health education is a still small voice. In the middle 1970s the tobacco industry spent 80 times more on advertising than the cost of all anti-smoking activities of government, and the alcohol industry 200 times more than health education on sensible drinking (King's Fund 1988: p. 88)[39]. Other governments might legislate for the 'knock for knock' policy used in the United States. This required that for every three tobacco advertisements on television, the tobacco industry had to pay for one health education advertisement (Whitehead 1989: p. 36)[40].

The cigarette and alcohol advertisers argue that their activities only influence choice of brand and not total consumption. But advertising does appear to influence children's consumption (King's Fund 1988: p. 78)[41]. The evidence from countries which have banned cigarette advertising has shown a reduction of mean annual consumption of 1.6 per cent a year while consumption has risen in countries with no controls by 1.7 per cent (Proctoscope 1991: p. 9)[42]. In Finland a complete ban on all forms of tobacco advertising led to a drop in smoking among 14-year-olds from 19 per cent in 1973 to 8 per cent in 1979 (Robson 1982: pp. 395–96)[43]. A particular problem is presented by the 300 hours of tobacco-sponsored sport on television (King's Fund 1988: p. 81)[44] and the advertisements at sporting events which cannot fail to be caught by the television cameras. It would be expensive and unpopular to buy out sport sponsorship by public subsidy and the obvious tactic of advertisers in response to bans on the appearance of their brand names on television is to diversify the use of the brand names, so that we are given Benson and Hedges wholemeal bread, Malboro margarine and Silk Cut muesli.

Conclusion

Changing people's lifestyles is far from easy. Health knowledge is not enough to change behaviour as people become prisoners to their social and economic environment. Vigorous action by government would help but the health lobby is seldom powerful except in Scandinavia. But the attitude among the public that it is the government's job to look after the nation's health and not theirs, is a strong obstacle. The fallacious repair shop attitude to health services, within which any damaged health organ can be patched up or replaced, breeds complacency. If people were led to recapture their responsibility for their own health, this attitude might change and so might the response of governments. But adverse material circumstances would still remain a major cause of unhealthy lifestyles.

Notes

1 Research Unit in Health and Behavioural Change (RUHBC) (1989), *Changing the Public Health*, Wiley, Chichester.
2 Foster, G.M. (1983), 'An introduction to ethnomedicine', in Bannerman, R.H. *et al.* (eds.), *Traditional Medicine and Health Care Coverage*, WHO, Geneva.
3 Foster (1983), 'An introduction to ethnomedicine'.
4 Foster (1983), 'An introduction to ethnomedicine'.
5 Koumare, M. (1983), 'Traditional medicine and psychiatry in Africa', in Bannerman, R.H. *et al.* (eds.), *Traditional Medicine*.
6 RUHBC (1989), *Changing the Public Health*.
7 Harwood, A. (1971), 'The hot-cold theory of disease: implications for treatment of Puerto Rican patients'. *Journal of the American Medical Association*, vol. 216.
8 Ankomah, A. (1992), 'Premarital sexual relationships in Ghana in the era of AIDS', *Health Policy and Planning*, vol. 7, no. 2.
9 Wellin, E. (1982), 'Implications of local culture for public health', *Human Organisation*, vol. 16.
10 RUHBC (1989), *Changing the Public Health*.
11 RUHBC (1989), *Changing the Public Health*.
12 Pearson, G. *et al.* (1985), 'Young people and heroin; an examination of heroin use in the North of England', *Research Report No. 8*, Health Education Council, London.
13 Amos, A. (1990), 'How women are targeted by the tobacco industry', *World Health Forum*, vol. 11.
14 'Round table' (1990), *World Health Forum*, vol. 11.
15 'Round table' (1990).
16 Macalister, M. (1992), 'The $225,000,000,000 habit', *Observer Colour Supplement*, 8 November.
17 Macalister, M. (1992), 'The $225,000,000,000 habit'.
18 Maynard, A. (1986), 'Economic aspects of addiction policy', *Health Promotion*, vol. 1, no. 1.
19 *Acquire* (1991), vol. 1, no. 1.
20 Smart, R.G. (1991), 'World trends in world alcohol consumption', *World Health Forum*, vol. 12.
21 Whitehead, M. (1989), *Swimming Upstream*, King's Fund Institute, London.
22 RUHBC (1989), *Changing the Public Health*.
23 Whitehead (1989), *Swimming Upstream*.
24 Whitehead (1989), *Swimming Upstream*.
25 Wallack, L. (1990), 'Two approaches to health promotion in the mass media', *World Health Forum*, vol. 11.
26 Wallack (1990), 'Two approaches'.
27 Macleod-Clark, J. *et al.* (1987), 'Helping patients and clients to stop smoking, phase 2: assessing the effectiveness of the nurses' role', *Research Report No. 19*, Health Education Authority, London.
28 World Health Organisation (1984), *Health Promotion: A Discussion Document on the Concept and Principles*, WHO, Copenhagen.
29 Levin, L.S. (1982), 'Life-style research and health promotion policy with special influence to mediating structures', (unpublished manuscript).

30   Dahlgren, G. and Whitehead, M. (1992), *Policies and Strategies to Promote Equity in Health*, WHO, Copenhagen.
31   Whitehead (1989), *Swimming Upstream.*
32   Whitehead (1989), *Swimming Upstream.*
33   Jones, E. *et al.* (1985), 'Teenage pregnancy in developed countries: determinants and policy implications' *Family Planning Perspectives*, vol. 17.
34   Jones *et al.* (1985), 'Teenage pregnancy'.
35   Smith, A. and Jacobson, B. (1988), *The Nation's Health*, King Edward's Hospital Fund for London, London.
36   Whitehead (1989), *Swimming Upstream.*
37   Wallack (1990), 'Two approaches'.
38   Wallack (1990), 'Two approaches'.
39   King's Fund (1988), *The Nation's Health.*
40   Whitehead (1989), *Swimming Upstream.*
41   King's Fund (1988), *The Nation's Health.*
42   Proctosope (1991), 'An obscene contradiction', *Times Health Supplement,* May.
43   Robson, J. *et al.* (1982), 'Sponsorship of sport by tobacco companies', *British Medical Journal*, vol. 284.
44   King's Fund (1988), *The Nation's Health.*

CHAPTER 4

Planning health policy

As shown in chapter 1, in countries at all levels of development the major determinants of health lie outside the health care system. Moreover, inequities in health are only likely to be radically reduced through actions involving such sectors as income distribution, housing, agriculture, education and environment (WHO 1986: p. 19)[1]. Planning for health needs not only to involve all sectors but all levels of government, employers, workers and communities. A distinction needs to be made between planning for health in its broadest sense and planning health services. Both are needed. Planning health services is the subject of Part Two.

Essentially any planning involves six steps:

- knowing where you are;
- deciding, quantitatively where this is possible, where you want to go and how to get there;
- deciding how far you can hope to get towards your target in a period of time (five or ten years);
- trying to get there in the time period;
- regular evaluation to see:
  – how far you have got,
  – where you are not on target,
  – how you can do better in the future;
- amending the implementation plan.

This approach is used by the World Health Organisation both at global level and at regional level. Once the Health For All programme was adopted in 1977, twelve global health targets were drafted and agreed in 1981. Progress towards these targets is reported to the World Health Assembly every three years and an evaluation is made in the following year. Similarly each region has produced its targets. Those for Europe were agreed in 1984. Each country is intended to follow with its own health plan and its own health targets.

The European targets which were endorsed by the countries are shown in Table 4.1. The classification develops one published earlier by the Canadian government (Lalonde Report 1974)[2].

In this classification, environmental factors are split between those put under 'prerequisites' and those under 'environment'. This was a political decision. While specific targets were agreed for all other headings, there were no targets for the prerequisites. It would have

Table 4.1   **Targets for Health for All 1984**

I.   Prerequisites for Health
     – Equity, minimum income, nutrition, peace, water, sanitation, housing,
       education, work, political will and public support

II. Lifestyle
     – opportunity
     – health promotion

III. Environment
     – hazardous conditions

IV. Appropriate care
     – priorities
     – primary health care

V.   Research
     – health knowledge

VI. Health development support
     – policy
     – management
     – education and training
     – technology assessment

Source: WHO (1986), *Targets for Health for All*, WHO, Copenhagen.

been very unlikely that all European governments would have agreed
to endorse such targets as full employment, adequate housing for all,
abolishing poverty or securing a minimum income for every citizen.
The list brings in the importance of research and support for health
development. And the whole list depends critically on political will
and public support. The key problems are that health development is
far from being the highest priority of many governments and the
public would resist certain attempts to make them healthy by passing
laws such as banning alcohol and tobacco. Nor would such laws be
enforceable without public support, as the experience of prohibition
showed in the United States in the 1920s. But the listing of the factors
affecting health assists in the process of creative thinking about some
of the measures of public policy which would favour health
development, if they were acceptable.

Planning health policy

This chapter sets out what a comprehensive policy for health would
look like. The central health problem in developing countries is
poverty. In 1989, over 30 per cent of people in developing countries
were classified as poor: in sub-Saharan Africa the proportion was just

under 50 per cent (Maxwell 1992: p. 7)[3], 15 per cent of babies are born underweight, 20 per cent of the population is anaemic and 8 per cent suffers from iodine deficiency (Maxwell 1992: p. 3)[4]. Poverty is also central to reducing health inequalities in developed countries. Beyond this the emphasis of policies diverges. This is because developing countries are faced with a high rural population and rapid population growth, and the focus must be on the health of mothers, children and those at work supporting families. Developed countries are much more urban and have low or negative population growth. Here the emphasis needs to be on the aged and on workers exposed to health risks: particular support needs to be given to promoting changes in lifestyles which endanger health.

In Table 4.2 are listed some of the methods and levels of intervention to improve health. In the discussion which follows, for convenience, action is classified by the government department concerned. While the lead may come from government, in many cases the success of the policy will depend on public acceptance and participation.

Table 4.2 **Forms of policy intervention**

---

1. TYPES OF ACTION
    Fiscal/monetary (incentives, subsidies)
    Regulation (economic, environmental)
    Direct provision (goods, services)
    Participatory guarantees
    Research/ development/ information/ education

2. LEVELS OF INTERVENTION
    National
    Local/community
    Household
    Material

3. LEVELS OF HUMAN ACTIVITY
    Physio/psychological
    Interpersonal/group
    Inter-group/inter-organisational
    Socio-political
    Ecological/environmental

Source: Milo N. (1986), *Promoting Health Through Public Policy*, Canadian Public Health Association, Ottawa.

Food and agriculture

A health-led policy would not simply aim to maximise production or maximise exports, but to ensure that food is available to provide a nutritious diet for the whole population. In a developing country, the well-being of the rural population depends upon adequate farm income and income from agricultural work, having enough energy for agricultural labour, protection from the health hazards of agricultural technology and the nutritional value of the food eaten. Food would be imported only where this is cheaper than producing it locally. Subsidies would be used to encourage the production and consumption of healthy foods and taxes to discourage the production and consumption of foods which are less healthy. An adequate diet would be made affordable by subsidies, land redistribution policies and/or by cash benefits. Home gardens and livestock are of particular importance for women in male-dominated societies since they can provide them with their own income.

At first sight, such a policy would reverse the priority for export-oriented crops in many developing countries. Land would be used to grow coffee, tea, cocoa, rubber and tobacco and other export crops only after the necessary land had been used to meet the population's nutritional needs. It is normally cheaper to satisfy these needs with traditional foods such as pulses, cassava, root and other vegetables and unpolished rice grown at home than by exporting crops and bringing in non-traditional foods from abroad. But some export crops can often generate much higher incomes, which can indirectly benefit the food entitlements not only of farmers but also of labourers and those dependent on non-farm sectors of the economy (Maxwell 1992: p. 7)[5]. But money from cash crops is usually controlled by men and a shift of food tastes to imported foods can lead to vulnerability from trends in market prices. New crops may not be as drought-resistant as old crops (WHO 1986: pp. 54–58)[6].

A variety of instruments can be used to develop a health-oriented policy in poor countries. They include pricing policies, state trading in staple foods, use of food reserves to stabilise prices, state subsidies for staple foods, feeding programmes for vulnerable groups, and routine fortification of suitable foods. In many cases food subsidies and feeding schemes have been of critical importance for vulnerable groups too poor to afford proper nutrition (WHO 1986: p. 68)[7]. A national child nutrition program would include growth monitoring, selective short-term supplementation and nutrition education. Such a program can be implemented through the primary health care system. In order to contain costs, the nutrition intervention program can be area-targeted (to regions having the highest child malnutrition rates), age-targeted (concentrating exclusively on children 6–36 months of age and pregnant and lactating women), and need-targeted. Targeting by need could be achieved by monitoring the weights of all children 6–36 months old in high malnutrition areas, and enrolling only those children whose weight gain over a certain period falls below standard. Those children would be singled out for special health monitoring, food supplementation and intensive nutrition education for their families (Berg 1987).[8]

But it is not only developing countries that need a national food policy. And adopting one depends on the willingness to act on evidence which is based on risk factors rather than on full scientific proof. The British government is to some limited extent prepared to act on such evidence in the case of alcohol and tobacco in the face of strong opposition from powerful industries. But it is less inclined to take on the agricultural interests. Britain is by no means the only country where the farming lobby is extremely powerful – often by holding the balance of power between the main contending political parties. Forcing some farmers to switch crops need not necessarily make the industry as a whole less remunerative, but it may well damage the interests of particular groups within the industry.

Risk evidence suggests that most of the developed countries consume an excess of dairy products leading to a high consumption of animal fats, inadequate roughage (wholemeal bread, root and green vegetables) and an excess of salt. Norway and Sweden have long been prepared to act on such evidence. The former has had a food and nutrition policy since 1975 but it has proved difficult to change farming and pricing policies in view of the strong lobby of the agricultural sector. Consumption of whole milk, cereals and margarine has followed the recommended policy but not consumption of sugar and potatoes (WHO 1986: p. 60)[9]. Japan, with the most favourable mortality experience in the world, has a major nutritional education programme.

Departments of agriculture have a special responsibility to control zoonotic diseases – those which can spread to humans through the food chain. Currently this is particularly important in developing countries. Irrigation can provide the right conditions for the breeding of mosquitoes that spread malaria; artificial lakes can lead to the proliferation of the snails that carry schistosomiasis; industrialisation can lead to the pollution of water with toxic chemicals, and the accompanying urbanisation can pose particular psychological hazards. It is therefore wise to incorporate preventive measures into industrial and agricultural projects which pose health hazards.

Tax policy

This is of vital importance for two reasons. First, the distribution of income is a key determinant of the health of populations. This can be changed by land redistribution and using the structures of both direct and indirect taxes. In developed countries, social security benefits play a major role in protecting the poor and redistributing income to those who are not at work. But they are often not sufficient to protect people from poverty in terms of the country in which they live. At the very least, the health sector can be used to help people claim all their entitlements. In developing countries, the limited ability to collect taxes limits the extent to which it is possible to finance benefits to protect the poor, but social insurance schemes covering those in regular work can be used to distribute cash benefits to those unable to work. The increasing tendency for developing countries to require parents to pay fees for primary education is a step in the wrong direction. Similarly user charges for health services are undesirable unless it is to ensure that supplies are sufficient in the health services to avoid sending patients to buy supplies (e.g. of drugs) in the private sector at much higher cost (see chapter 12 below). What is paradoxical is that many of the countries moving in the direction of fees and user charges spend heavily on defence, even where there is no obvious enemy in sight. Where general subsidies or cash benefits cannot be afforded to help the poor, policies can at least be developed to provide nutritional help in kind to vulnerable groups such as undernourished infants and school children. Food subsidies or similar interventions can be introduced but they can be very expensive and, unless very carefully chosen, benefit the rich more than the poor. They cost over 10 per cent of gross domestic product in Mozambique and 7 per cent in Egypt (WHO 1986: p. 9)[10].

Second, as mentioned earlier, tax and subsidy policy can be deliberately used as a health promotion strategy to encourage or discourage consumption on health grounds. It has been established by a number of studies that increasing the price of cigarettes does reduce tobacco consumption. For example, an increase in price of 1 per cent would cut consumption in the United Kingdom by 0.5 per cent (Atkinson and Townshend 1977: pp. 492–95)[11]. The effect is likely to be greatest in the lower income groups where smoking is more prevalent. In Papua New Guinea the effect would be larger – 0.7 per cent (Chapman and Richardson 1990: pp. 537–40)[12]. Part of the tax revenue can be used for health promotion as has been done in Victoria, Australia and in Finland and Iceland (Dahlgren and Whitehead 1992: p. 14)[13].

On the other hand, while in 1964 it took a manual worker in Britain six hours to earn the price of a bottle of whisky, by 1984 it took only two hours (King's Fund 1988: p. 88)[14]. This could have been prevented by higher taxation. Whether reducing licensing hours, or abolishing them in the attempt to make visits to the pub a family outing, would increase or reduce alcohol consumption is not established.

The use of taxation could be carried further by taxing vehicles according to safety. Thus motor cycles would be very heavily taxed, followed by three-wheel vehicles and then cars according to their accident rates. Healthy foods, low alcohol drinks and facilities for exercise could be subsidised from taxes on unhealthy foods and alcohol. For example, there could be a tax based on the animal fat content of foods. Already lead-free petrol is sold at a lower price than leaded petrol in many developed countries and this has led to its widespread acceptance.

Environmental and housing policy

First, there are the issues which are either global or international such as deforestation, acid rain, nuclear risks, the disposal of toxic chemicals and the pollution of rivers and dams. Preventive action involves costs within countries while many of the benefits of action would be enjoyed by other nations. This is an international issue and thus requires international action on which, so far, there has been little or no agreement.

Second are the largely internal issues of which safe water and sanitation are the most obvious. Nearly half the population of developing countries suffers from health problems associated with unsafe water and inadequate sanitation (WHO 1986: p. 101)[15]. Infant and childhood diarrhoeas are estimated to cause 4.5 to 5 million deaths a year out of 600–700 million episodes. It is estimated that improved water and sanitation could cut morbidity by 25 per cent (WHO 1986: p. 102)[16]. Increased availability does not necessarily ensure increased access or increased utilization. What is vital is close community involvement in such projects from the planning stage onwards (WHO 1986: p. 104)[17].

Housing should be adapted to local climatic and environmental conditions. Like animal shelters and food storage facilities, housing needs to be proof not only against the elements but also against insects and rodents that carry disease. All these structures, and particularly kitchen and sanitary facilities, should be easy to clean and cooking stoves need to be carefully designed to avoid children suffering serious burns. Most developed countries have the taxable capacity to ensure that every family has a decent home and a variety of strategies are used to go some way to making this possible in many countries in Europe. This is not practicable in developing countries. But the policy of building showers and WCs on plots of land and leaving the family that rents the plot to gradually build round the sanitary facility with what materials it can afford is a step to improving the health of lower-income families even if it does not reach the poorest. The orientation of policy should be to assist communities and families to build for themselves. Health-related policies include upgrading slums and shanty towns by the provision of basic amenities and the legal recognition of squatter settlements.

Housing has many health aspects: safety from fire and earthquakes, adequate internal space, heating, safe places for children to play and the undesirability of using materials which cause health problems – whether it is the use of woods which harbour insects in developing countries, or concrete which causes condensation in developed countries. Regulation can be used to enforce minimum standards in developed countries. In developing countries, they may make the position of the poorest worse and not better: regulations can impose costs which are beyond the reach of the poor (WHO 1986: p. 125)[18]. If it is not possible to provide safe places for children to play, at least it is possible to slow down traffic by 'sleeping policemen' in streets where children play if there is no alternative.

Labour

First, there are the physical health risks of work which vary enormously between different occupations. Mining, fishing and construction work are particularly hazardous. The aims are to promote safety, prevent occupational diseases, and protect children from employment which will endanger their health. And they can be enforced by legal sanctions and a strong inspectorate. What is important is that employees are alerted to health risks. In many countries trade unions play an important part in pressing for healthy working conditions. At the very least the costs of industrial accidents should be made to fall on employers though a scheme of workers' compensation.

Second, there are the stresses and psychological effects of work processes. It is particularly stressing where the pace of the work is set by the conveyor belt and the work is divided up into monotonous repetitive tasks.

The workplace can be a very effective setting for health promotion and promoting worker participation in such activities as restricting smoking opportunities and promoting sport and leisure activities.

The evidence is now overwhelming that unemployment is health-damaging. In many developed countries a gap has arisen between the types of skill which employers are seeking and those possessed by the unemployed. Thus vacant posts for skilled workers remain unfilled while there is large-scale unemployment. Programmes of training for the unemployed and for women seeking to re-enter the labour market are health-promoting. Countries with a heavy emphasis on occupational training, such as Germany, Switzerland or Sweden, have less unemployment. What is critical is to reduce the risk of unemployment among those with a weak position in the labour market, including disabled people. An active labour market policy is part of inter-sectoral action for health.

Transport

Travel on railways is much safer than travel on the roads. Yet many countries provide and maintain free roads from taxes but expect railways to pay their way. Transport policy should do the reverse. Where toll roads are impracticable, road costs should be recovered from taxes on fuel. But road safety will remain a problem. This can be promoted by, for example, seat belt and crash helmet laws, vehicle inspections and pedestrian protection. Learner motorcyclists can be restricted to lower-powered motorcycles as in Australia (Johnson

1992: p. 155)[19]. Drunken driving can be reduced by random breath testing. Safety, including skid-resistant road surfaces, should be an important consideration in road construction. Cycle tracks need to be provided in all city roads as in Denmark and the Netherlands. No-smoking areas need to be steadily increased to all public transport and public offices and no smoking regulations on aeroplanes as well as buses extended. The aim should be to make healthy living an easy option and thus to encourage more people to choose it.

Education

As pointed out earlier, female literacy is of crucial importance for health by starting to teach the logic of scientific thought. Only a few years at school can provide basic skills and some capacity for continued learning. Mothers notice a child's illness at an earlier stage and gain the confidence to take action, whatever old relations may say. There is also a close relationship between educational levels and the acceptance of family planning (WHO 1986: pp. 77–79)[20]. Non-formal education of adults has also been used, for example, to promote the use of oral rehydration in a relatively short period.

But schools provide enormous opportunities as centres for providing health care to the young and as focal points for community health. Schools should be made deliberately health-promoting. Meals at school can be provided by rotas of parents as in villages in Thailand. On top of this, schools can provide health promotion at the formative period of life. The content should include not only attitudes to the use of tobacco, alcohol and drugs, but hygiene, nutrition, exercise, and sex (even more critically important in view of the AIDS epidemic). Health education at schools can have an influence on parents, particularly when they can become involved. It is a means of introducing behavioural changes and basic health concepts into the homes of pupils. Success depends on teacher training, appropriate teaching and learning materials and the development of clear goals.

Health

The first requirement is to ensure that health facilities are available all over the country. Urban concentration is not only a problem in developing countries. Finland created new posts for doctors in the rural areas of Lapland and Eastern Finland by 70 per cent subsidies from the central government. The average salary in a health centre was considerably higher than in the hospital sector (Dahlgren and Whitehead 1992: p. 43)[21].

Home visits by health visitors, public health nurses, and voluntary health workers can increase home safety and increase the take-up of immunisation services. After a visit from a health visitor in England giving specific advice on how to reduce the hazards in their homes, 60 per cent of parents took steps to improve the safety compared with 9 per cent who were only encouraged to look at a programme on television on home safety (Colver *et al.* 1982: pp. 1177–80)[22]. Where health visitors spent an hour a month with parents, immunisation rates rose to 90 per cent compared with 50 per cent in other comparable areas (Barker and Anderson 1988)[23]. An alternative is to use community health workers working with groups of mothers in poorer areas and helping them to identify their felt needs and to address their health concerns. By starting with the life situation of those it is planned to help and assisting them to build up the confidence to feel that they can change their lives in a number of respects, the impact is likely to be more lasting. It is, however, difficult to evaluate such projects.

Health inequalities

Action should be deliberately planned to give priority (including extra resources) to those facing the most serious health hazards, at home and at work, and those most deprived. In developing countries, this may mean concentrating action in areas or districts with the lowest agricultural production per household, the poorest rates of school attendance, the highest indicators of malnutrition, or living in the worst slums. In developed countries income, social class or rates of unemployment can be used. Special efforts can be made to improve take-up rates for immunisation and other preventive care (including family planning), if necessary by home visits, and to improve the accessibility and quality of local health services. These visits can also be used to give specific advice on home safety and hygiene. Where possible the extent of take-up should be monitored. Extra health education in schools and school meals can be provided in deprived areas and efforts made to improve sub-standard housing and reduce pollution. In developed countries primary health care centres can be used for debt counselling, job training and advice on how to claim every type of social security benefit. But what is needed most of all is less unemployment, better housing for the poorest with easy access to nurseries, health facilities and shops and an absence of pollution, an improvement in the worst working conditions and less inequality of incomes (Dahlgren and Whitehead 1992)[24].

Taking inter-sectoral action seriously

One possible list of interventions to improve health is shown in Table 4.3. The actions are classified according to the framework of the European Health Targets.

Table 4.3 **Some possible interventions to improve health**

PREREQUISITES
Create greater income equality by:
  – high progressive income tax,
  – food subsidies,
  – high taxes on luxury goods,
  – minimum income from social security
    paid for by lower defence spending;

Greater emphasis on female education

Provide water and sanitation or, in a developing country, materials for communities to build and maintain the facilities;

Subsidise housing for the poor;

Employment policy – paid work for all who want it with crèches for mothers with young children.

ENVIRONMENT
Reduce accidents by:
    – seat belts, motor cycle helmets, safer road construction, safer cars, speed limits, pedestrian crossings etc,
    – control of sale of consumer goods with risks for children,
    – occupational safety;

Fine those who pollute the atmosphere, rivers, etc.

LIFESTYLE
Heavy taxes and controls on advertising of cigarettes and alcohol;

Subsidise healthy foods, tax unhealthy foods;

Public health nurses visiting homes;

Mass media and health educators, community health workers.

APPROPRIATE CARE
Promote primary health care with community participation

This is by no means an exhaustive list, but by indicating some of the fields for inter-sectoral action it points up the breadth of a healthy public policy. It challenges traditional economic thinking by suggesting that the value of production cannot be simply measured in terms of average dollars per head but in terms of its contribution to the health and happiness of the citizen. Such a policy cannot be promoted by a health ministry acting alone.

Action of this kind depends above all on the determination of government as a whole to make it happen. Support is needed at the centre of power. A number of developing countries accepted the broad scope of 'Health for All' policies and established new governmental machinery to handle it. For example, within three years Sri Lanka established a National Health Council chaired by the Prime Minister. It included the ministers responsible for health, agriculture, education, finance (and planning), local government, home affairs, labour and rural development. Its functions were to give leadership to health development, guide and coordinate the ministries, and create community awareness, participation and involvement. It is serviced by a committee of the senior civil servants concerned. Beneath it are district health councils for each of the 24 administrative areas of the country (Marga 1984)[25].

In Thailand, the Social Development Project was established under the National Economic and Development Board to coordinate action by four key ministries – Agriculture, Education, Health and the Department of the Interior. Basic minimum needs indicators were established for identifying gaps at the village level for priority action. These included hygienic nutrition, adequate shelter and environmental conditions and the development of pre-school children. The resultant 'quality of life indicators' were incorporated in the Sixth National Development Plan (WHO 1986: p. 36)[26].

Within a year of the publication of the European health targets, Sweden established by a parliamentary resolution an Inter-sectoral Health Council with officials from the departments of labour, housing, agriculture, transport and public administration. It already had a National Road Safety Office. The coordination of health promotion became the responsibility of the health education division of the National Board of Health with a staff of 25, consisting of behavioural, educational, political and social scientists: none of them were doctors. In 1985, it published a health plan for the 1990s (National Board 1985)[27] and hosted, in association with WHO, an international conference on inequalities in health and health care (Nordic School 1985)[28]. In 1991, all public agencies and authorities were required by parliament to report on specific goals to reduce inequalities in health (Dahlgren and Whitehead 1992: p. 12)[29].

Australia established an Australian Institute of Health and Welfare (AIHW) with representatives from the relevant departments plus representatives of consumers of health services, housing assistance and welfare services and an expert in public health research. Its task is to monitor the progress of health and welfare policy, press for the reorientation of training and new priorities in health research and encourage community participation[30].

Within the Japanese Ministry of Health, there is a division of health promotion and nutrition whose budget has been increasing many times faster than that of the whole ministry. There are 17 Regional Health Promotion Centres concentrating on nutrition, physical fitness and relaxation exercises to relieve stress. Underneath the Regional Centres are 670 Local Health Promotion Centres. There are 150,000 trained nutrition volunteers. Of the roughly 3,000 municipalities in Japan, by 1984, 91 per cent had established Local Health Creation Councils to coordinate the health policies of different ministries at the local level. On top of all this, all health insurance societies in Japan, which finance the curative health services, are required by law to spend 5 per cent of their budget on preventive activities. They finance health counselling, regular physical fitness checks, health seminars, sports events, health exhibitions, food preparation courses and newsletters. In addition they train health opinion leaders. Not until 1989 were the corresponding German sick funds, on which the Japanese health system was originally modelled, allowed by law to spend money on health promotion (Abel-Smith 1992: p. 26)[31].

By contrast, the British government did not respond to the 'Health for All' policy for seven years after the European targets were endorsed (DoH 1992)[32]. And even then, no priority was given to health inequalities.

Conflicts of public policy

The key problem is that health promotion is by no means the only aim of public policy. Promoting exports and the jobs at stake at home are very influential considerations with politicians. The European Commission wants to ban tobacco advertising but subsidises growers by £1.5 million a year. Both tobacco and alcohol are major export earners for Britain. For example, the United Kingdom has three of the world's seven largest tobacco companies and is one of the seven largest producers of tobacco in the world. With exports of cigarettes to 150 countries, net exports of £309 million in 1991 and a contribution of £8 billion to the exchequer in VAT and duty (Macalister 1992)[33], the industry provided 20,000 to 40,000 jobs in no less than 60 parliamentary constituencies (Cadman 1984: pp. 285–88)[34]. The British government refuses to ban tobacco advertising because to introduce a statutory advertising ban 'on a product which is legally for sale is a very serious step to take in a free country'[35]. Restrictions on tobacco imports by developing countries are viewed by the United States government as an impediment to free trade. The alcohol industry generates an estimated 125,000 jobs directly or indirectly (King's Fund 1988: p. 58)[36]. And both industries are contributors to the funds of political parties. It is sometimes suggested that the loss of tax revenue from tobacco and alcohol would be a major concern to governments but it could readily be replaced by a higher value-added tax. But in some developing countries, the potential loss of export revenue from tobacco is a serious consideration. Compared to the lobbies behind these two giant industries, the pro-health lobby is weak, divided and poorly organised both at national and local level.

Conclusion

The above examples show that some nations do take health policy seriously, attempt to coordinate it at both the national and local levels, and develop community participation in action to promote health. The most resolute action seems to be taken in countries which already have very good health indicators as judged by expectation of life.

Notes

1   World Health Organisation (1986), *Intersectoral Action for Health*, WHO, Geneva.
2   Government of Canada (1974), *A New Perspective on the Health of Canadians* (The Lalonde Report), Queen's Printer, Ottawa.
3   Maxwell, S. (1992), 'Food security in Africa', *Africa Recovery*, no. 6, September.
4   Maxwell (1992), 'Food Security'.
5   Maxwell (1992), 'Food Security'.
6   WHO (1986), *Intersectoral Action*.
7   WHO (1986), *Intersectoral Action*.
8   Berg, A. (1987), *Malnutrition: What Can be Done? Lessons from the World Bank Experience*, Johns Hopkins, Baltimore.
9   WHO (1986), *Intersectoral Action*.
10 WHO (1986), *Intersectoral Action*.
11 Atkinson, A.B. and Townshend, J.L. (1977), 'Economic aspects of reduced smoking', *Lancet*, vol. 3.
12 Chapman, S. and Richardson, J. (1990), 'Tobacco excise and declining tobacco consumption: the case of Papua New Guinea', *American Journal of Public Health*, vol. 80, no. 5.
13 Dahlgren, G. and Whitehead, M. (1992), *Policies and Strategies to Promote Equity in Health*, WHO, Copenhagen.
14 Smith, A. and Jacobson, B. (1988), *The Nation's Health*, King Edward's Hospital Fund for London, London.
15 WHO (1986), *Intersectoral Action*.
16 WHO (1986), *Intersectoral Action*.
17 WHO (1986), *Intersectoral Action*.
18 WHO (1986), *Intersectoral Action*.
19 Johnson, I. (1992), 'Action to reduce road casualties', *World Health Forum*, vol. 13, no. 2/3.
20 WHO (1986), *Intersectoral Action*.
21 Dahlgren and Whitehead (1992), *Policies and Strategies*.
22 Colver, A. *et al.* (1982), 'Promoting children's home safety', *British Medical Journal*, vol. 285.
23 Barker, W. and Anderson, R. (1988), 'The Child Development Programme: an evaluation of progress and outcomes', *Evaluation Document No. 9*, Early Childhood Development Unit, Bristol University.
24 Dahlgren and Whitehead (1992), *Policies and Strategies*.
25 Marga Institute (1984), *Inter-sectoral Action of Health*, Marga Institute, Colombo.
26 WHO (19896), *Intersectoral Action*.

27 The National Board of Health and Welfare (1985), *The Swedish Health Services in the 1990s*, Liber Trych, Stockholm.

28 The Nordic School of Public Health (1985), *Inequalities in Health and Health Care*, Goteborg.

29 Dahlgren and Whitehead (1992), *Policies and Strategies*.

30 See *AIHW News*, Canberra.

31 Abel-Smith, B. (1992), *Cost Containment and New Priorities in Health Care*, Avebury, Aldershot.

32 Department of Health (1992), *Health of the Nation*, Cm. 1986, HMSO, London.

33 Macalister, M. (1992), 'The $225,000,000,000 habit', *Observer Colour Supplement*, 8 November.

34 Cadman, M. (1984), 'The politics of health: the case of smoking control', *Journal of Social Policy*, vol. 13, part 3.

35 Statement by Mrs Virginia Bottomley to the House of Commons Health Select Committee on 28 October 1992.

36 King's Fund (1988), *The Nation's Health*.

PART TWO

Planning health services

CHAPTER 5

The history of the organisation and financing of services

Modern scientific medicine has a history of not much more than two hundred years. Indeed it has often been said that it was not until the twentieth century that the average patient who consulted the average doctor was likely to derive benefit from the encounter. Nevertheless, effective remedies for some illnesses were developed in Europe in the nineteenth century and earlier and some preventive action came to be taken, if not always, from a correct understanding of the process by which illness spread. This is not to deny that schools of medicine in other parts of the world, such as China or India, had developed effective remedies earlier.

Long before there was effective medicine, those who could afford it visited doctors and were purged, bled and provided with a range of distasteful medicines. The effective medicines developed in the nineteenth century, other than laxatives which were used in excess, included morphine, quinine, strychnine, atropine and later codeine and cocaine. It was not until the end of the century that X-ray and pathology came to be used as diagnostic tools. Until the development of anaesthetics in the 1880s, only quick and superficial surgery could be practised – cutting out stones in the gall bladder, lancing of boils, removing cataracts and amputations. As modern scientific medicine gradually proved its value, it steadily reduced the role of traditional medicine which had evolved in Europe as elsewhere.

The development of hospitals

Those who had comfortable homes stayed in them when they were sick. But hospitals came to be provided in many different cultures. They were found in the Indian culture and in the huge Arab kingdom which spread across Southern Europe, as well as in the early Christian Church. Hospitals became part of monasteries and convents and various sisterhoods and brotherhoods had duties to care for the sick. During the thirteenth century there were some 19,000 hospital units or annexes in Europe (Commission on Hospital Care 1947: p. 426)[1]. Hospitals served the sick who were without families or servants – the poor, the travellers and those working away from home. Special provision was often made for soldiers and sailors for whom government accepted a duty of care. But a further need, increasingly recognised during the nineteenth century, was to isolate those with infectious diseases, although the precise methods by which infections were spread were little understood. Thus hospitals were created for smallpox, cholera and typhoid. During the nineteenth century, special public hospitals were established in Sweden to treat cases of venereal disease in hospital and in Norway to isolate lepers. Hospitals were also set up to confine mental patients of all social classes who were seen as a danger either to themselves or others or both.

Gradually, or suddenly in the case of the French Revolution, many continental hospitals were transferred from control by the Catholic Church to control by public authorities because of either mismanagement, misappropriation of funds, anti-clericalism or just the absence of adequate financial backing (Burdett 1890: pp. 76, 423, 454, 618)[2]. In Spain and Portugal and their colonies in Latin America, however, the Catholic Church retained a major role in the provision of hospitals until well into the twentieth century.

By 1870, it had been made the duty of local authorities to provide hospitals in both Denmark and Sweden (Burdett 1890: pp. 448–57, 662)[3]. Thus, in Scandinavia, the hospitals were developed largely as a public service. Indeed the Swedish hospitals were separated from the poor law during the eighteenth century and came to be regarded, early on, as a service provided for the whole community. They were originally provided by the smallest units of government (the parishes) and financed by a head tax. From 1862, the hospitals were handed over to the newly formed counties and financed from taxes on spirits and charges to patients (Anderson 1972: pp. 39, 42)[4].

In Britain, after Henry VIII had suppressed the monasteries in 1536, such hospitals as there were became secular institutions. Charitable bodies provided the bulk of acute hospital care until the National Health Service was established in 1948. But this private sector was gradually supplemented by public provision for the mentally ill, under the poor laws for the chronic sick and cases of infectious disease, and from the 1930s for acute cases where provision was inadequate. From the early nineteenth century, the majority of the physically ill in institutional care were in publicly owned institutions and gradually special and separate provision was made for them (Abel-Smith 1964)[5]. It was accepted that most patients were unable to pay. Patients' direct payments never contributed much to the running costs of hospitals. It was not until 1881 that any major hospital accommodated paying patients at all.

The British system of charitable hospitals was extended to North America (Commission on Hospital Care 1947: p. 434)[6]. But there was also a long tradition of small private hospitals set up by physicians or surgeons for their own patients. From the early days, the charitable hospitals took a substantial proportion of paying patients: by 1893, the majority of hospital beds were occupied by paying patients in the United States (Commission on Hospital Care 1947: p. 442)[7].

The extensive development of government and charitable hospitals in Europe for those who could not afford to pay led to the appointment of doctors to work in them – generally, in the case of public hospitals, for a full-time or part-time salary. Thus there emerged a separate class of paid doctors with hospital appointments. This higher class of doctors obtained a virtual monopoly of the principal hospital appointments which provided them with the opportunity to specialise. In Britain, the leading doctors worked in the charitable hospitals without payment and supported themselves by the consultations of private patients. It increasingly became medical etiquette for these specialists to confine themselves to cases referred by general practitioners (Abel-Smith 1964)[8]. Those who could not afford to see a specialist on a private basis were seen in the outpatients' departments of the charitable hospitals. Similarly, in Sweden extensive outpatient departments were developed in the local authority hospitals.

Care for the poor outside hospital

In a number of countries of Europe, the poor law or social assistance services paid doctors on a part-time or full-time basis to look after the poor. In Norway salaried doctors to care for the poor have a history of over 350 years (Burdett 1890: p. 56)[9] and similar systems were developed in Poland, Sweden and Switzerland and the United Kingdom, from 1818 in one of the States of Germany (Nassau) (Sigerist 1941: p. 142)[10] and from 1864 in Russia.

Midwifery developed as a separate free-standing profession in Britain, the Netherlands, France, Belgium, Germany and some other countries. Salaried midwives came to be appointed in Britain to attend the births of the poor. Though opposed by the medical profession, midwives became officially registered from 1902. In the United States medical opposition to this development was successful. Home nursing was started as a separate charitable movement in Britain from 1859 and in time came to be heavily subsidised by and gradually transferred to local authorities.

Developments in the colonies

In Latin America one of the first initiatives of the colonisers was to provide a high standard of hospitals for the armed forces and later for the police. These hospitals for those who administered 'law and order' have generally survived to the present day. In addition both the Spaniards and the Portuguese endowed a limited number of Catholic hospitals (*beneficencia* or *santitas casas*) which were supported by the wealthy to relieve distress among the poor. Small payments were made to the medical staff for their part-time services. As the cost of providing hospitals increased, many of them received grants from government to augment their incomes from charitable sources. These Catholic hospitals were later supplemented by government hospitals, health centres and medical posts staffed by part-time salaried doctors – particularly where there were no charitable hospitals. When employers established large enterprises far from the towns to exploit natural resources, they also established health services. Later laws were passed requiring large employers operating far from the organised services to establish specified health services. Such a law was enacted in Peru in 1924.

When Europeans developed colonies in Asia and Africa, hospitals and other health services were originally provided only for the army and for the colonists. In time, these services were extended on a limited basis to the indigenous population, but mainly in the urban centres. Environmental health services were also started and campaigns to combat the main infectious diseases. In some colonies (e.g. India) the government hospitals were supplemented by indigenous charitable efforts and in many by mission hospitals – particularly in Africa. As in Latin America, where large mines and plantations were established far from the towns, employers began to provide medical services and legislation was often introduced requiring them to do so.

Voluntary insurance

Meanwhile, a strong voluntary health insurance movement had developed in Europe, out of which compulsory health insurance was later to develop. Organisations of working men, often developing out of the guilds, pioneered the system. Mutual benefit societies under a variety of names (such as friendly societies and sick funds) were established from the late eighteenth century as industry developed and a class of working people, separated from the land, formed in the towns and cities. This sickness insurance movement was often run by local workers for their mutual benefit and was strongest among the more skilled workers. Contributions were generally a flat rate sum per week, though there were variations in the benefits for which members could subscribe.

In 1804, about 30 years before the British Medical Association was formed, there were about a million members of friendly societies in Britain in a population of some 10 million. Originally they provided cash benefits in sickness. but later doctors were engaged to certify sickness and provide treatment. By 1900, there were some seven million members of societies which were officially registered and probably several million more in unregistered societies – most of them entitled to invalidity cash benefits, the services of doctors and the drugs they prescribed. Development was similar and on almost the same scale in the Netherlands and Denmark. Small farmers as well as workers joined as members. As clubs of local people everyone paid the same rates or premiums there were no attempts at risk-rating, though someone with obvious long-term illness might be excluded from joining in the first place.

The voluntary sickness insurance movement was also extensively developed in Austria, Germany and Switzerland during the nineteenth century (Newsholme 1931: p. 241)[11]. The movement spread later to Australia and New Zealand though on a smaller scale. While in Northern Europe, the schemes were based on local areas, in central Europe they were generally based on employers. The employer often contributed and in the course of time contributions became a proportion of earnings. A further difference is that the Northern European schemes did not normally cover hospital care as this was not seen as a high priority and the charitable or public hospitals were already making provision. Hospital care became more often covered in central and later Southern Europe.

There were many ways of securing the provision of services. Some used what the International Labour Office classifies as the direct method – professionals were salaried and the fund built and organised the facilities where the services were provided. This pattern was particularly likely to be chosen where services were underdeveloped. Often the direct method was opposed by health professionals, arguing that this challenged professional freedom, though what was often feared even more was the loss of economic freedom. Others used the indirect method: existing local providers were contracted. More often than not the doctor was paid on a capitation basis – a monthly sum for each member whether that member had cause to use the service or not. This simplified administration for these small voluntary societies and made it easier to predict expenditure. Part of the membership fee was set aside for the doctor and part for the cash benefit. In the early days doctors were expected to provide the drugs out of their capitation payment.

Thus, particularly in Northern Europe, consumers of medical care came to be organised before the doctors were effectively organised, and they were in a position to dictate the terms of service for the doctors whom they engaged. The doctors were servants to the funds. There were many aspects of the terms of service which caused resentment. The societies tended to appoint some doctors and not others: those excluded found many of their patients were induced to transfer to the doctor who was appointed (Hogarth 1963: p. 211)[12]. Disciplinary matters were handled by lay committees. And finally, the level of remuneration was regarded as grossly inadequate. It was by no means uncommon for a society to put the job out to tender, though they did not necessarily always give the post to the doctor who offered to do it for the lowest price. What was particularly resented was where patients who could well afford to pay the normal private practice fees of the doctors were members of the societies. The resentment of the doctors led them to develop new medical organisations or to strengthen existing ones to fight the societies (Abel-Smith 1963: p. 20)[13].

One strategy of the doctors was to try to organise boycotts of those societies which were considered to be paying their doctors too little. All doctors were told not to apply for the appointments they advertised. But this was never very successful in Europe; some doctors simply defied the boycott. However this tactic did work in Australia, where the societies in Victoria simply had to close in 1918. They were only able to start up again in 1920 when they conceded a stated level of capitation payment, the right to charge extra for operations, and an income limit for membership. A second tactic was to try to persuade the registering authority to rule that working for a society was 'unethical' for a doctor. This tactic failed in Europe. The third strategy was for the profession to establish its own societies which operated on the principles they favoured and try to attract members from the older societies. This approach was more successful but the doctors never managed to secure a majority of the membership of societies (Abel-Smith 1988: pp. 694–719)[14].

Voluntary health insurance was also started in Argentina, Brazil and Uruguay though later and on a much smaller scale. In Latin America its function was to secure better services than were provided by charity for immigrants of particular nationalities. In the United States, consumer-run friendly societies with contracted doctors were started on the European pattern in a number of cities before the First World War, but the medical profession was successful in killing off this development. County medical societies ruled that it was unethical for doctors to contract their services with an organisation of this kind. From 1929 a number of cooperatives were started in the Western States despite strong opposition from the medical profession. By 1949, there were over a hundred cooperatives but ten years later only a handful were still functioning. By that time, Blue Cross and Blue Shield were dominating the health insurance market – both sponsored by the providers.

Compulsory health insurance

Meanwhile, building on the voluntary precedents, the first compulsory health insurance scheme was started in Germany in 1883. Indeed compulsory insurance had been pioneered for civil servants in some of the states that were to form Germany from the eighteenth century. But the major precedent was the mines. Medical care had been provided to miners in several states from the sixteenth century. Some employers employed their own doctors and provided their own small hospitals. The miners contributed to the health insurance fund and the employer generally contributed a share of the profits. Increasingly, these schemes became regulated by laws specifying the obligations of employers and making contributions compulsory.

By the early nineteenth century, Prussia had laws which not only regulated provisions for miners but for civil servants as well. After the revolutionary year of 1848, a law was passed allowing municipalities to order workers to join mutual welfare funds which provided medical care and other benefits. Employers could be made to contribute up to 50 per cent of their workers' contributions and became represented in the administration of the fund. This legislation was also enacted in other states later on and by 1868 there were over half a million members of some 4,000 funds in Prussia alone (Abel-Smith 1966: pp. 13–14)[15].

Thus the law of 1883 had many precedents. One motive was to cut the cost of poor relief. But the main one was to contain socialist and revolutionary pressure by creating a new loyalty of workers to their employer and the State. The chancellor, Bismarck, who introduced the law wanted the scheme to be run by the State to strengthen loyalty to it. He was, however, over-ruled by the legislature which insisted that the schemes should continue to be run by employers and employees. The scope of the law was gradually extended until all lower-paid workers were required to join a fund.

It was not long before the government became involved in disputes between the sick funds and the profession concerning levels and methods of remuneration, disciplinary sanctions and other matters. The major protests from the doctors were about the 'closed panels' of doctors selected by the sick funds. They demanded the right for any doctor to work for the funds. The substitution of payment per case and later fee-for-service for capitation payments or salary, which the profession fought for and eventually won, was a means of establishing open competition between all doctors who wished to take part in health insurance work.

In Britain, compulsory health insurance also involved the extension of an existing system – that of the friendly societies, many of which had by this time become large and politically powerful national organisations. Lloyd George, the architect of the 1911 compulsory scheme, had studied the German system but he adapted it to British precedents. His motives were narrower than those of Bismarck. While he was concerned about the health of workers, after so many had been rejected as unfit to fight in South Africa, he also wanted to rescue workers from the unpopular poor law services and at the same time reduce its cost. But his main concern was to win popularity with the working class and gain greater support for the Liberal Party at the expense of the growing Labour party. The announcement that there would be a scheme galvanised the British Medical Association into action, demanding what it had long failed to persuade the friendly societies to concede – higher remuneration, an income limit for membership, the right for any doctor to participate and representation in the management of the scheme. Virtually all these demands were met. Thus while the intervention of government in Britain rescued general practitioners from friendly society control, in Germany it initially enhanced the power of the sick funds over the profession.

Compulsory insurance was steadily developed in the other European countries. Some abandoned any income limits for membership. The capitation system of payment, and the closed panels associated with it, were eliminated in Norway and their role substantially reduced in Denmark, Italy and Austria. Where fee-for-service payment was used, this generally had the effect of fragmenting the delivery of care between episodes of illness as patients shopped around and tried new doctors, particularly specialists. But capitation was still used in much of Denmark, the Netherlands and Britain, and in the rural areas of Italy and Spain. It had the effect of protecting, promoting and crystallising the concept of the general practitioner as the doctor to whom the patient went first for medical care.

Whether provision for hospital care was covered by health insurance varied among the European countries. Where hospitals had developed as a government service as in Scandinavia, or on a part government and part charity basis as in Britain, they continued with this financing and charges for them were eventually abolished. Where contributions were a proportion of earnings shared with the employer, as in most of continental Europe, the cost of hospital care was included in the scheme, so that both local authority and private hospitals had their negotiated charges paid direct by the health insurance funds. This led to a rapid expansion of doctor-owned small hospitals (*cliniques*) in France. There was a similar development in Japan.

Elsewhere, the poorly developed hospital system was supplemented by new hospitals built by the social security agency itself as in Spain and parts of Italy. This became the predominant pattern of development in Latin America, where compulsory health insurance schemes were developed from the 1920s onwards. Where there were separate social security funds for separate occupational groups, each fund built its own hospitals; in some countries the funds competed with one another in the lavishness of their provision. Existing hospitals were, however, normally used by the schemes started in India (1948), Burma (1954) and Tunisia (1960). These schemes started on a small scale, but the Indian one was to grow and cover over 30 million persons.

In the 1920s, opposition to doctors being paid direct by health insurance schemes developed in France. The medical profession did not want the German system of health insurance imposed upon them. It was held that the doctor should be paid direct by the patient and not by a 'third party' – government, social security or private insurer. The doctors refused to participate in the government's health insurance scheme unless it operated on a reimbursement basis. This was finally conceded in 1929 and the patient was reimbursed 80 per cent of a negotiated fee. The crucial point was that this left doctors free to charge more than had been negotiated on their behalf and governments ever since have sought to restrict or limit this practice, with only temporary success (Bridgman 1971: p. 333)[16]. Similar systems were adopted in Belgium, in Australia from 1930 and later in Canada from 1962. The opposition to third party payment became a critical policy stance of the profession in the United States from the 1920s. When compulsory health insurance was finally introduced, after many attempts, but confined to the elderly from 1966 ('Medicare') not only was reimbursement used, but there was not even a negotiated schedule of fees until 1993: doctors could charge what was 'reasonable', taking into account their customary charge and the prevailing charges of other doctors in the area. This was almost a unique arrangement: the only other cases under a compulsory scheme were the Philippines and Taiwan.

The extension to universal services

Once most of the regularly employed were covered, the problem facing policy-makers wanting to extend rights to health care was how to cover the self-employed – particularly farmers, fishermen and others, many of whom had relatively low earnings and no employer to share the contributions. One solution was to keep the cost of insurance down for all insured persons by providing highly subsidised public hospitals of acceptable quality as in Scandinavia. Another was to make the other funds cross-subsidise the low-income self-employed. A third was to subsidise all compulsory health insurance with public funds or only certain funds for the self-employed. Many ways have been devised to try to collect some contribution from farmers – taxes on land according to its potential profit (as in Italy), taxes on agricultural produce (as in Brazil) and contributions collected as part of the income tax, in the knowledge that farmers were well-placed to understate their incomes (as in the Netherlands, France and Belgium).

The final stage of development has been services available to all. Hungary attempted this briefly in 1920 and the former Soviet Union greatly extended the government-financed services established under the tsars to cover the whole population by 1938. Britain was the first Western European country to follow in 1948, then Japan and Scandinavia in the 1960s, Canada in the 1970s, Italy in 1980, Portugal, Brazil and Spain in the 1980s, and South Korea in 1990 with Taiwan planned for 1994. (It should however be added that health insurance of different kinds has a very high coverage in the other Western European countries.)

How did countries with insurance-based systems make the

transition to services available to the whole or nearly the whole population? Usually those not covered included the unemployed, the aged, and the disabled. Some countries covered the aged as dependents of insured persons. Others built rights to health care on to cash benefits, given as part of their social security schemes. Thus people receiving benefits for sickness, disability or unemployment, or pensions for widowhood or old age were deemed to have prepaid, while they were at work, for cover to health care to be continued while they were on benefit or pension. Or a modest contribution was taken from the pension while it was in payment. Those on social assistance had their contributions paid for them by the central or local government agency which provided the assistance (Glaser 1991: pp. 37–38)[17].

Three important points should be made about this stage of development:

1. Countries generally retained their previous arrangements for the provision of services.

The United Kingdom was exceptional in choosing this moment (1948) to take nearly all its hospitals into central government ownership.

2. Most countries retained health insurance contributions as one of the sources of finance for the universal services.

How far they did so depended on the balance decided upon among different ways of raising money for public services, taking account of ease of collection and the side-effects on the operation of the economy. An exception is Denmark. A partial exception is the Netherlands, where social security contributions are collected as part of the income tax but still separately labelled. But this option is not available in countries with poorly developed income tax systems.

3. Whether the system of universal health provision was called a 'national health service', 'national health insurance' or 'national health system' was simply a question of political choice.

Not surprisingly the term 'health insurance' was retained in such countries as Japan, Korea, and Canada where the use of the term a 'national health service' might sound socialistic. Nor is it surprising that the term 'national health service' was preferred by some left-of-centre governments and by the right-wing government of Italy when it depended on the left to keep it in power. The Scandinavians have been much more relaxed about nomenclature. They see no more advantage in talking about a national health service than of a national education service. Both are seen largely as the routine functions of local government, like providing fire services.

Countries which have not developed universal services have chosen not to do so for a number of reasons which need to be appreciated. The attempt failed in the Netherlands in the 1970s because of opposition from the trade unions, but another type of universal scheme may come into effect in 1995, as described in chapter 15. The trade unions realised that their members would have to pay more for their health services if everyone was covered on the same basis. Providers would no longer give their members favourable terms if they could no longer make high charges to the higher income groups who were covered by voluntary insurance. This consideration operates to some extent in Germany. But there is also the fact that many of the high income groups with low health risks who are excluded from health insurance can buy private health insurance cheaper than if they were forced to pay a contribution related to their earnings. There is also a problem when there are many different funds. None of them may want to take in uninsured people, who, it is feared, will include high health risk persons who are currently a burden to social assistance services and not to sickness funds.

The only developed country without extensive compulsory health insurance is the United States. It was restricted to the aged, was introduced as late as 1966, and gave very incomplete coverage. Provision for the poor was left to the individual states and the extent of it became very variable. Free or highly subsidised health care were long provided to the poor in Europe before compulsory health insurance was established. Europe also had the precedent of a large coverage of voluntary health insurance supported by the workers and the consumer movement. The United States did not have the same precedents. After consumer-sponsored health insurance had been virtually eliminated by concerted action by the medical profession, voluntary health insurance was developed by providers, not con-sumers, and later profit-making insurers entered and dominated the market. This meant that premiums were related to risks and varied by size of employer and could not be afforded by many small employers. Nearly 40 million people had no health insurance at all and many more had inadequate coverage. The United States became the odd man out among the developed countries because of attitudes to the poor and their association with 'blacks' and new immigrants, the lack of development of a strong and united trade union movement and the power of the medical profession to use a political system which responded to strong lobbies.

Meanwhile, many ex-colonies in Africa and Asia greatly extended the free or nearly free health services which they had inherited from the colonisers. More hospitals were built, expatriate doctors were replaced by those locally trained, and the attempt was made to extend services into the rural areas. To a varying extent these countries made use of auxiliary health workers. The services remained exclusively financed from taxes and it was not long before the ambitious aim of providing free or nearly free services to the whole population came face to face with the problem of limited taxable capacity. The problem became acute in the early 1980s when the economic crisis destabilised the economies of the developing world.

Conclusion

Underlying the different provisions for health care are differences of national values and differences in the political influence of different actors – doctors, trade unions, employers and consumers. Health care has always been regarded as more of a right in Western Europe than in the United States. The attitudes of the latter influenced Latin American countries with their substantial indigenous population, though the trade union movement was able to secure compulsory health insurance for the more powerful groups of workers.

Notes

1   Commission on Hospital Care (1947), *Hospital Care in the United States*, The Commonwealth Fund, New York.
2   Burdett, H.C. (1890), *Hospitals and Asylums of the World*, vol. 3, Churchill, London.
3   Burdett (1890), *Hospitals and Asylums*.
4   Anderson, O.W. (1972), *Health Care: Can there be equity?*, Wiley, Chichester.
5   Abel-Smith, B. (1964), *The Hospitals 1800–1948*, Heinemann, London.
6   Commission on Hospital Care (1947), *Hospital Care*.
7   Commission on Hospital Care (1947), *Hospital Care*.
8   Abel-Smith (1964), *The Hospitals*.
9   Burdett (1890), *Hospitals and Asylums*.
10 Sigerist, H.E. (1941), *Medicine and Human Welfare*, Yale, New Haven.
11 Newsholme, Sir A. (1931), *International Studies on the Relations between Private and Official Practice of Medicine*, vol. 2, Allen and Unwin, London.
12 Hogarth, J. (1963), *The Payment of the General Practitioner*, Pergamon, London.
13 Abel-Smith, B. (1963), 'Paying the family doctor', *Medical Care*, vol. 12.
14 Abel-Smith, B. (1988), 'The rise and decline of the early HMOs: some international experiences', *Milbank Quarterly*, vol. 66, no. 4.
15 Abel-Smith, B. (1966), *Value for Money in Health Services*, Heinemann, London.
16 Bridgman, R.F. (1971), 'Medical care under social security in France', *International Journal of Health Services*, vol. 1, no. 4.
17 Glaser, W.A. (1991), *Health Insurance in Practice*, Jossey Bass, San Francisco.

CHAPTER 6

Methods of health service planning

The aim of health service planning is to improve the health of the population. Health for All principles require priority for those whose health is most disadvantaged. All planning has to be conducted within limited resources. This is a fact of economic life. Thus, in theory, any public resources devoted to health services should aim to achieve the maximum health benefit for the resources spent – particularly for those whose health most needs to be improved.

There are three difficulties in implementing this principle. First, as pointed out early in the first chapter, health is not a one-dimensional concept. There are different elements of health. Blaxter listed them as disease, disability, frequency of illness, malaise and fitness. Second, even if weights could be agreed on for the relative importance of these different dimensions of health, there would still remain the problem of fitting survival into the picture. What importance, for example, is attached to prolonging survival even if that survival is clouded by disease, acute disability and severe pain? Should a year in this state be counted as 10 per cent or 50 per cent of a year in good health? Third, epidemiological knowledge on the effectiveness of health interventions is limited. What, for example, would be the difference in the incidence of measles if 60 per cent of children were immunised compared to 80 per cent. While for some conditions, an outright cure can be predicted, for others there may be only a temporary improvement in functioning. What importance should be attributed to this? Similar is the difficulty of establishing how far the use of more sophisticated diagnostic tools actually improves outcome. Finally, there are political considerations. For example it would not be acceptable to provide no treatment for diabetes because the lifelong treatment for it is expensive.

The difficulty of measuring the output of health services makes it difficult to fit health plans into national plans for all sectors, which tend to be dominated by economic considerations. The economic planners tend to respond to demands where the output of capital expenditure can be quantified. Thus plans for infrastructure developments tend to be given priority over plans for health development. The extent to which better health improves productivity, and how much the long-term investment in human capital contributes to output and lower birth rates, cannot be so easily established. Planners can too easily assume that expenditure on health services is simply current consumption which takes resources away from investment in agriculture and manufacturing (Wheeler 1985: p. 193)[1].

Despite all the intrinsic difficulties, it is better to plan than not to plan. This is because of the obvious waste and distorted priorities which can arise in an unregulated private market. If planning can go some way to check waste and redirect priorities, the endeavour will have been worthwhile. But the starting point should be a modest recognition of the limitations of what planning can be expected to achieve.

An unregulated health market

An unregulated health market leads to waste because of the peculiarities of the demand and supply for health services. The health market is practically unique in the lack of mechanisms for self-regulation. Consumers want health but often do not know what they need to do to get it, other than seek professional advice. Doctors may know what patients need but have no incentive to see that it is provided economically – whether they are providing it or acting as a purchasing agent. Some restraint operates when patients have to pay the bill out of their own pockets. But when the patient has taken out insurance and all the insurer does is to reimburse costs in whole or part, as many insurers do in the United States, even that restraint is partly removed. Where doctors own health facilities, they are faced with conflicts between their entrepreneurial role and their professional role. The supply of hospital beds, as explained in chapter 10, generates within limits the demand for hospital beds. Doctors can enter over-doctored areas and provide unnecessary services, leaving other areas devoid of medical personnel. Competition in the health market can lead to unnecessary surgery, excessive diagnostic tests, excessive prescribing, as well as overuse of hospitals. It can also lead to poor quality in other ways such as a lack of specialisation of skills and a lack of regular practice in undertaking delicate procedures.

Doctors and dentists possess monopoly rights conferred by law and are reluctant to delegate. Once the doctor writes a prescription with a brand name, normally the pharmacist has no right to substitute a cheaper product. The doctor has allowed the price to be fixed mainly by the monopoly manufacturer of that product. Even where a generic is prescribed, the patient is unlikely to spend the time shopping around for the lowest price. Moreover, pharmacists are reluctant to become cut-price salespeople.

There is no single organisation pledged to secure the best service at the best price. The market is fragmented and each part is out to make a profit if there is no effective countervailing power. Such a private market cries out for regulation, and planners can do much to rationalise the system without having to come to grips with the contentious issue of priorities. In a public health system, giving in to pressure groups may lead to too many doctors and two few paramedicals.

The purposes of health planning

Planning is needed to prevent waste, make full use of scarce resources, contain costs to what is affordable and see that they are distributed geographically on an equitable basis. In many countries, planning is, in effect, a rationing process. Though guidelines may come from the centre, plans should be built up by aggregating and reconciling local plans. At the local level planning may be combined with the task of managing. At the central level a separate group is usually assigned to construct the plans after consultation with those responsible for different parts of the service. Planning may not be confined to the public sector but extend to the regulation of the private sector.

It is easy enough to state the objective of health planning, but such a statement only obscures some of the difficulties. Ideally health planning aims to secure that necessary services of the right quality are provided at the right place at the right time, that the health services have a balanced relationship with other social services, and that this is achieved at the lowest possible cost in real resources and is affordable by the country concerned. Necessity is a question of degree: priorities specifying what is most necessary will vary according to what a country can afford. There is a tension between quality, which in some contexts requires specialisation and therefore geographical concentration, and local availability. Obviously not all services can be available everywhere on a 24-hour basis, though transport to services can be. The term 'lowest cost' raises the question of whose costs – the balance between the time and travel costs falling on patients and relatives and the costs falling directly on the services.

Finally it should not be forgotten that plans affect many interest groups – the professions, the committees that run hospitals, administrators, trade unions, local politicians and the local users of services. Those who work in the services do not normally want their work disturbed and the public normally wants services kept where they are used to finding them. Economic interests will also often be at stake. Thus changes in services, however 'rational', are likely to encounter opposition and obstruction. For these reasons, there is a strong temptation for planners not to disturb the status quo. If there is more money for the health system, it tends to be distributed on much the same basis as existing expenditure, on an 'incrementalist basis'. While this is hardly a theory of planning, it is a good description of what, in practice, many countries actually do. Some plans consist of no more than a list of proposals for capital expenditure on separate projects in the government health services (Wheeler 1985: p. 201)[2].

Methods of planning

There have been a number of attempts at fully comprehensive 'rational' planning and systems of such planning have been taught to health planners. Rational planning 'demands full knowledge of all alternative courses of action, full knowledge of all causes and effect relationships and complete agreement on the goals to be pursued' (Lee and Mills 1982: p. 48)[3]. Two examples are presented below to show the limitations of approaches of this kind.

Health service planning in the former Soviet Union

The basic assumption underlying the use of the system developed in the Soviet Union was that all health 'needs' could and should be met by the organised health services. Thus the first step was to measure the extent of health need. Massive surveys of up to one and a half million people, which included medical examinations, were mounted to obtain this data (Hilleboe *et al.* 1972: p. 38)[4]. Populations were screened to see what health care they 'required'. How much of this morbidity was preventable? And what resources would be needed to take this preventive action? How far would such action reduce need in the future? Forecasts were made of future changes in income, environment, morbidity, population structure, population movement and other factors (Popov 1971: p. 46)[5]. Having estimated future need, the next step was to quantify the resources needed to meet it.

This was calculated by convening the appropriate specialists to reach a consensus on such questions as what drugs would need to be prescribed, whether referral to a specialist would be necessary, what diagnostic tests should be undertaken and, if admission to hospital was required, how many days the patient should stay and what procedures would need to be undertaken during the stay. The end product of the whole planning system was norms. A basic norm was that a consultation with a primary care doctor needed 20 minutes and that a nurse needed to be present during the consultation. There were similar norms for visits to specialists. And the results of the epidemiological surveys were used to calculate the ratios of different categories of doctors, nurses and auxiliaries needed per 1,000 population; the drugs, equipment, disposables and the number of hospital beds needed per 1,000 population. By the late 1960s patients in urban areas were visiting doctors nearly 10 times a year and using 9.3 beds per 1,000 population (Popov 1971: pp. 52, 69)[6].

Using this methodology, local plans could be developed on the basis of local demographic patterns. What gaps remained to be filled in terms of the capital stock of buildings and equipment? What was the deficit in terms of trained health workers? What further resources were needed in terms of supplies?

Finally, five-year plans could be produced showing how much of the shortages could be made good in the next planning period, given the extra economic resources which were planned to be made available for the health sector. Then a detailed plan was made for the next year.

At first sight, the system seems to have an unassailable logic. There are, however, fundamental snags. First it is assumed that demand is the same as medically determined need. Perceived need and medically determined need are very different concepts and it is the former which determines the demand for health services. In all societies a large amount of medically determined need is dealt with by self-care and care within the family. Second, it assumes that all health need can be medically determined, which is not the case. Some very real illnesses cannot be proved to exist by any medical tests. Third, it assumes that it will at some stage be economically possible to meet all medically determined need at the norms for the use of resources laid down. This was never achieved in the Soviet Union: resources were spread very thinly over the country except in the case of certain prestige facilities reserved for senior officials or key industries. Health-trained personnel were not in short supply but were not always well trained and the modern equipment which they needed to function was often lacking.

Finally, and this compounded other failings, the use of norms built a static bias into the system. There was no, or inadequate, provision for technological change. While primary care doctors in England and Germany were seeing patients on average for six minutes without a nurse present at the consultation, the 20 minute norm remained in force in the Soviet Union. While lengths of hospital stay were falling drastically throughout the world, as a result of new drugs, improved diagnostic equipment and procedures, tests done before admission and the recognition of the importance of early ambulation after surgery, the Soviet Union remained conservatively bound by cosy norms which gave the staff a quiet life. Just as the industrial system continued to produce old-fashioned goods by old-fashioned methods, so the health care system became locked into old wasteful ways of treating patients, long since replaced in the West.

The PAHO/CENDES system

This methodology was developed from 1961 by the Pan American Health Organisation (PAHO) and the Centre for Development studies (CENDES) in Venezuela. It was long taught in planning courses throughout Latin America. Unlike the Soviet system, it did take account of limited resources. It was based on a simple economic proposition. 'A resource is efficiently used if the benefit obtained from its use is greater than that which would have been obtained if the same resource had been used for something else' (Alumada *et al.* 1965: p. 6)[7]. The principle is fine in theory. The difficulty comes in applying it. Recognising the difficulty of obtaining useable data on morbidity or disability, the planning system became based exclusively on mortality.

Thus it became a system of calculating which deaths could be prevented at lower cost. The underlying aim became to maximise the number of deaths prevented out of a given budget.

That this should be the sole aim of the health system was a massive value judgement which would be unlikely to secure the assent either of the doctors, who in theory were to operate it, or of the public and the politicians representing them. Should there be no treatment at all provided for conditions which are very disabling but do not cause death? Would the doctors or the public accept such explicit priorities? If the deaths which could be prevented at low cost were all concentrated in a limited number of regions of the country, would it be acceptable for all health effort to be concentrated in these regions, and nothing to be provided in the other regions, even though the main finance for the health sector was drawn from the more prosperous regions which did not have any of the deaths cheapest to prevent? Presumably because of all these difficulties, the logic of the method was modified by adding that the existing level of care of diseases that cannot be reduced would be retained (Alumada *et al.* 1965: p. 16)[8].

The methodology also assumed that the information to operate the system, if not already available, could be assembled at reasonable cost. Clinical trials to attempt to obtain all this information would be considered far from ethical. Also, the process of calculating costs is not without its problems. To give just one example, some health outputs are jointly produced and need to be jointly produced to make efficient use of resources. How can the costs of particular interventions be isolated? But the most important assumption underlying the methodology is that health planning is a rational process which can readily be left to experts (economists, epidemiologists and others) to work out the details, and that any recommendations will readily be implemented by the politicians. Any methodology founded on this assumption is flawed at the very root.

For all these reasons, though the CENDES methodology was taught throughout Latin America for at least 20 years, it was never really applied in practice. Health planners became buried in the task of trying to make sense out of inadequate statistics and had little influence on what was happening, particularly in countries, such as much of Latin America, where the health sector is dominated by social security schemes which have their own dynamic and priorities, outside the reach of ministries of health.

The cost-benefit approach

A less ambitious attempt to establish broad priorities is by looking at the costs and benefits of a limited number of frequently used interventions. Finding an acceptable way to measure the benefits of health services is inevitably controversial, as pointed out earlier in this chapter. The World Bank uses disability-adjusted life years in its 1993

World Development Report. By this criterion, it shows that primary health care interventions are very cost-effective in reducing childhood malnutrition and mortality, mainly from infectious diseases. Also very cost-effective, but given insufficient attention, are chemotherapy against tuberculosis, integrated prenatal and delivery care, mass programmes to de-worm children, condoms plus information and education to combat AIDS and measures against smoking (World Bank 1993: p. 61, fig. 3.2)[9].

At first sight this may imply that where health resources are limited, all effort should be directed at these objectives and less cost-effective interventions should not be provided at all. Such a policy would not, however, be politically acceptable. But the value of this type of calculation is to show which common interventions should be given greater priority within a system of primary care. The obvious field for reducing expenditure so that more can be spent on these interventions within primary care is to limit the role of tertiary hospitals to that originally intended for them, for reasons given in chapter 10 below.

Practical planning

If plans are going to be implemented, they must have political backing and the support of those for whom the services are being planned. Hence the need to involve the community in the planning process at every level. One great advantage of the 'Health for All' initiative of the World Health Organisation, endorsed by most countries of the world, is that health planners in each country can start by assuming that ministers of health are serious in wanting to implement these priorities, though they may compromise when they see the full implications.

The World Health Organisation's recommendations on planning follow the six basic principles set out in chapter 4. The recommended structure of planning is set out in the managerial process for national health development shown in Table 6.1.

The first stage is to select broad priorities in the light of the current situation and national development goals. These are then developed into strategies with, where possible, quantitative targets – broad programming. In detailed programming the resources needed to achieve the objective are estimated. Then the programmes are implemented and, finally, evaluated and the lessons learnt are used to revise the programme.

Evaluation is intended to be carried out by those providing the services, those using them and those responsible for managerial control at the different levels of the service. It has several parts. First, it is necessary to re-examine the relevance and priority of the programme. Second, the actual progress has to be assessed. Third, the efficiency has to be evaluated by comparing the results achieved with

Table 6.1   **Managerial process for national health development**

PROGRAMME BUDGETING EDUCATION		INFORMATION SUPPORT
	HEALTH RELATED SOCIO-ECONOMIC SYSTEMS	
	FORMULATION OF NATIONAL HEALTH POLICES	
	BROAD PROGRAMMING	
	DETAILED PROGRAMMING	
	IMPLEMENTATION	
	REPROGRAMMING	

Source: WHO (1980), *Guiding Principles of the Managerial Process for National Health Development*, WHO, Geneva.

the resources used. Fourth, the effectiveness of the outcome has to be considered.

So the first step is to make decisions on what most needs to be changed – on where you want to go. A new minister of health may arrive with a clear mandate indicating what changes he or she wants made. The senior staff of the ministry may try to sell ideas to the minister. Or the planner may remind the minister of the WHO's broad priorities for equity, primary health care and community participation. A determining factor may be what appears to be most susceptible to change. Once decisions are reached on the broad strategy, the planner works out in detail the implications in terms of resources (buildings, staff, supplies and money). At this stage constraints may be identified which determine the possible pace of change. Or the minister may make a judgement on what is politically possible in view of likely opposition. Then a detailed policy can be drafted. It should start with a description of the current situation (knowing where you are) – how all health resources are distributed both geographically and in terms of expenditure on primary and secondary/tertiary care and other programme structures, relevant to the chosen strategy. A number of such structures are shown in Table 6.2.

Table 6.2. **Possible programme structures**

TARGET GROUPS
  Age and sex, Income level, Social class, Ethnic group, Geographical area

FUNCTION OF SERVICES
  Prevention, Treatment, Promotion, Rehabilitation, Support

LEVELS OF CARE
  Primary, Secondary, Tertiary

BROAD DISEASE PROBLEMS
  Malaria, Diarrhoeal diseases, Tuberculosis, AIDS etc.

CLIENT OR DIAGNOSTIC GROUPS
  Mentally ill, Mentally handicapped, Aged, Children, Pregnant Mothers etc.

CLINICAL SPECIALITIES
  Surgery, General Medicine etc.

DEGREE OF DEPENDENCE
  Nursing and social support needed

Source: Adapted from Lee and Mills (1982), p. 89

Further structures are, of course, possible. But by no means all countries would be able to document the current situation of expenditures on all the different dimensions shown in the table. A plan which attempts to operate on many different dimensions at the same time is likely to be too difficult to implement in practice. Those in the field need to be given very clear objectives, and not too many of them, on which they can focus their attention and know that they will be judged by the proven progress they make on those particular objectives.

The objectives should then be turned into guidelines for local planning, setting out the main objectives, the levels of health care to be aimed at in terms of types of unit, their equipment and staffing to serve different populations. There should also be indicators of performance and efficiency including unit costs (Segall 1991: p. 61)[10]. Then local planners should examine their existing health services according to these guidelines and prepare their plans accordingly. The plans are then added together and tested for affordability, as discussed in chapter 16.

Etzioni called this type of process 'mixed scanning' (Etzioni 1967)[11]. The analogy is a wide-angled camera which would cover the whole landscape but not in great detail. A second camera would zoom down on those areas indicated by the first camera as worthy of a more in-depth examination.

Policy instruments

Regulation to move towards planning objectives can be applied to the whole health care system (public and private) or only to the public sector (whether financed by taxes or compulsory insurance contributions or some mix of the two). Often much stronger regulation is applied to the public sector with the aim of limiting public expenditure.

The main methods of regulation can be classified under the following headings:

Budget control

In directly controlled services, the management can, at least in theory, impose chosen priorities on the system by budgeting, central direction or specifying specific targets to be achieved by particular services. But there are limitations. Instructions given are not always carried out, and trained staff have many ways of resisting appointment to unpopular places – including ultimately leaving the service. Even in such systems, it is helpful to reinforce directives with financial and other incentives.

Budgets can be imposed on hospitals or on the whole of a publicly financed health care system. Budgets can be used to subsidise the construction of more facilites in under-provided areas. Budgets can drive more of the funding year by year in the desired direction – for example, towards primary health care or selected preventive activities. Or budgets can be imposed on different parts of the health system or types of hospital to assert priorities.

Regulation through purchase from the private market

This can consist of the negotiation of prices and/or the methods of paying for services, The payment system may be selected because it limits incentives for extra services and/or gives incentives for particular types of service. The prices set may aim to make some priority types of service more profitable than others.

Regulation of supply

The common field of application is on the number of hospital beds. Additions or extensions are required to have central approval or they will not be recognised as providers when it comes to payment. Or when the payer owns the beds it uses (such as a public health service), it can apply local norms in deciding what to provide. Similarly, the installation of major medical equipment can be made subject to prior approval or directly rationed. But increasingly it is recognised that the number of hospital beds needed depends on the extent of provision of alternative modes of care – in institutions or at home. Thus planners may stimulate the provision of these alternatives.

A second common field where supply can be regulated is the work-force – doctors (separating general practitioners from specialists), dentists, nurses and paramedicals. Production can be made subject to central control and incentives given for doctors to train in unpopular specialties. Moreover incentives can be given to try and secure that existing trained personnel are located in response to need.

In many developing countries, moving towards greater geographical equity and a greater priority for primary health care and specific preventive services are seen as sufficient objectives for the immediate future. The move to primary health care in itself involves asserting priorities through the essential principles of primary health care defined by WHO as set out in chapter 8 below.

Securing compliance

There are limits to what can be achieved by regulation or paper planning. The private sector has its own, often competing objectives. And in some poorer countries substantial power is exercised by external donors and international agencies which have their own agendas that may differ from those of the government. Plans may encounter opposition from the medical profession and the political elite who favour priority being given to urban hospitals providing highly specialised care (modelled on those in developed countries) and opportunities for private practice. Some professional policy-makers may favour the interests of their own groups (Walt and Vaughan 1986: p. 46)[12].

Plans may also encounter opposition from powerful local interests. To be effective, planning often resolves into a process of negotiation. There is always a tension between the desire of the centre to have its way and the need for local flexibility and discretion. What is important is that those who are to carry out the plan come to 'own' the objectives. One way of trying to create this situation is by starting planning at the lowest level of the administration ('bottom-up planning') so that the administrators at this level have to prepare their own plan, given certain guidelines. Motivation and participation increase where people feel they are in a position to influence decisions which affect their lives. But it is still difficult to get acceptance of a plan where it challenges strong local interests. Failure to focus attention on local acceptability and prepare a strategy for 'selling' the plan is the most common cause of failure in implementation.

Examples of the use of different forms of regulation to achieve planning objectives are given in the chapters which follow.

Two examples of plans

Zimbabwe

The newly independent government inherited in 1980 a health care system heavily oriented towards the urban areas and towards curative care and divided into two separate services of very different standards – one for whites and one for blacks. Rural health facilities were severely damaged, under-supplied and under-staffed as a result of the war. In the capital, Harare, infant mortality was 14 per 1,000 among whites and between 30 and 50 among blacks. It was estimated as 140 per 1,000 in rural areas rising to 200 per 1,000 in the most deprived areas. Only about a fifth of babies were born in rural areas in institutional care; the maternal mortality rate was as high as 145 per 100,000 births even in government maternity units. Among the most important causes of death of children were diarrhoea, pneumonia, measles, tetanus, malaria and tuberculosis. Only about a tenth of the rural population had access to safe water and sanitation.

The main objective of the government in its health plan published in 1984[13] was to give priority to primary health care in a context of community involvement and democratisation. This meant rebuilding (or repairing) and restaffing facilities, the training and reorienting of health staff (particularly using village health workers), giving a positive role to traditional practitioners and securing adequate drug supplies. The distribution of finance was to be used to enforce these priorities. Health was to be integrated with other fields of development. Specific targets were laid down for immunisation, water and sanitation, infant, child and maternal mortality, ante-natal care, malnutrition and so on.

The Netherlands

Many of the themes set out in the European Health for All programme – such as reducing inequality, the emphasis on promotion and prevention, the stress on community participation and the critical role of primary care – were already widely accepted in the Netherlands. The task was to translate these themes into specific policies and do so in a context where efficiency was critical, as costs had to be contained. A national steering committee on future health scenarios was set up with sub-committees to look at specific important health problems. For each policy issue, past trends were analysed and effectiveness of existing action was assessed before scenarios were developed for future development. These reports were widely disseminated and discussed.

Targets were defined for each policy issue, where possible in quantitative terms. For example, mortality from ischaemic heart disease in persons under age 65 was to be reduced by 30 per cent.

Conclusion

These two examples of planning bring out some common themes. Neither tried to plan everything at once. In both cases particular priority problems were identified and the plan was designed to deal step by step with those problems. In both cases targets were laid down – how far it was hoped to make progress towards desired objectives within a designated period.

No plan is likely to be fulfilled exactly as specified and the assumptions, particularly the economic assumptions, underlying the plan are likely to change in the course of time. As a result any plan will need regular revision. Thus in practice most plans end up as being rolling plans: every year or two the plan for the next five to ten years is re-specified.

The quality of planning depends upon the quality of information used for making the plan and the skill of the planners. It also depends on regular evaluation of why past plans have failed to be successfully implemented.

Notes

1 Wheeler, M. (1985), 'Health sector planning and national development policy', in Lee, K. and Mills, A. (eds.), *The Economics of Health in Developing Countries*, Oxford University Press, Oxford.
2 Wheeler (1985), 'Health sector planning'.
3 Lee, K. and Mills, A. (1982), *Policy-making and Planning in the Health Sector*, Croom Helm.
4 Hilleboe, H.E. *et al.* (1972), *Approaches to National Health Planning*, WHO, Geneva.
5 Popov, G.A. (1971), *Principles of Health Planning in the USSR*, WHO, Geneva.
6 Popov (1971), *Principles of Health Planning*.
7 Alumada, J. *et al.* (1965), *Health Planning: Problems of Concept and Method*, PAHO, Washington D.C.
8 Alumada *et al.* (1965), *Health Planning*.
9 World Bank (1993), *World Development Report 1993: Issues in Health*, World Bank, Washington D.C.
10 Segall, M. (1991), 'Health sector planning led by management of recurrent costs; an agenda for action-research', *Health Policy and Planning*, vol. 6.

11   Etzioni, A. (1967), 'Mixed scanning: a third approach to decision-making', *Public Administration Review*.

12   Walt, G. and Vaughan, P. (1986), 'Politics of health planning', *World Health Forum*, vol. 7.

13   Government of Zimbabwe (1984), *Equity in Health*, Government Printer, Harare.

CHAPTER 7

Planning the health work-force

The aim of planning human resources for health is to secure that the right mix of skills with the desired orientation is available in the right place and that this is achieved with minimum waste. The mix of skills which is appropriate for a country will depend on long-term plans for development of the health services.

In not a few countries, the human resources which have been trained are a major factor determining what health services are provided and where they are provided. In other words, the tail wags the dog. For example, surgery is more practised in the United States than in Britain because there are more surgeons. Throughout the world, some areas have good services and others poor services because health professionals want to practise in some areas and not others. Primary care is under-developed in some developed countries because most doctors want to be specialists and are trained as such. In many developing countries, primary care is under-developed because doctors will not work in remote rural areas and not enough paramedicals have been trained who will. Where standards of public health are poor, it is often because few doctors want to enter this field of medicine. Low standards of care for the mentally ill and mentally handicapped are partly due to the fact that these are neither prestigious nor popular specialities.

The theme of this chapter is that the right balance of skills will not occur without careful planning because of the conflicts between economic forces, political pressures and professional objectives. Thus it is important to understand the forces which have led to the present situation.

Simple comparisons between countries show the extent of imbalance in the production and deployment of human resources trained for the health field. Some extreme examples are the following (Bankowski and Fulop 1987: pp. 18, 25, 26, 62)[1]:

- While there were 276 doctors per 100,000 population in Czechoslovakia and 249 in Belgium, there were only 6 in Benin and 1 in Ethiopia.
- While there were three to four nurses to one doctor in some Northern European countries, there was one nurse to two doctors in Argentina and five doctors to one nurse in Pakistan.
- There were 100 times more nurses per head in Canada than Pakistan.

- While there were over 40 dentists per 100,000 in Argentina, Brazil and Canada, there was only 1 in India and Pakistan.
- In Greece, nearly two-thirds of doctors were specialists while in the United Kingdom just over a third were specialists.
- In Italy, comparing the provinces, there were twice the ratio of doctors in urban provinces than in rural provinces. In Brazil the ratio is three to one and in Senegal twenty-seven to one.
- In 1978, doctors in Thailand were distributed so that 73 per cent were in Bangkok where only 9 per cent of the population lives (Roemer 1988: p. 547)[2].

The world doctor surplus

World-wide, there is an immense over-production of doctors. Some of the estimates of the surplus of doctors in 1987 and the projected future surplus are shown in Table 7.1. The definition of surplus doctors differs from country to country. In some of them, the medical association keeps a register of doctors seeking jobs, though these doctors may or may not be doing a small amount of private practice and an occasional locum. In some others, a committee has reviewed the situation and projected the surplus from the extent of current under-employment among doctors. In some cases the surplus has to be calculated from the number on the register of doctors compared with the number known to be in practice. Doctors working abroad and retired doctors cannot be separated in the figures.

The table is far from giving the whole picture as data for many countries were not available. Only a few Latin American countries are included. But it is estimated that three-quarters of Latin American countries already have a doctor surplus (Roemer 1988: p. 54)[3]. Moreover, while there were, in 1987, 295,000 doctors in Latin America and the Caribbean, there were in the same year some 300,000 medical students. In view of all this data, it would seem that the year 2000 will be celebrated with a world surplus of some quarter to half a million doctors.

The current surplus is also partly due to the emphasis given by WHO in the 1950s and 1960s on the need to produce more doctors. Many developing countries set themselves targets of the ratios of doctors per 1,000 population which they aimed to achieve. There was a rapid expansion in medical schools, particularly in developing countries, as shown in Table 7.2. The increase was three times faster in the developing countries than in the developed. The annual rate of increase in developing countries was about 60 times greater than in developed countries. (Bankowski and Fulop 1987: p. 19)[4].

It would seem likely that the surplus of doctors will be followed by a world surplus of dentists. Since the 1940s the prevalence of caries and periodontal disease has fallen remarkably. It is estimated that the

Table 7.1 **Estimated doctor surplus**

Country	Surplus in 1987	Projected surplus for the year 2000
Canada	800	5,000+
USA	?	150,000
Sweden		7,000
Norway		3,200
Denmark		2,300
Finland		3,400
Germany	29,399[1]	Rising?
Netherlands	2,500	Rising?
Spain	23,000	Rising?
France	20,000	Rising?
Italy	45,000	Rising?
Japan		16,000–64,000
Pakistan	6,000	21,000
Bangladesh	5,000	Rising?
Egypt	4,000	Rising?
Korea		26,500
Mexico	39,193	Rising no quota
India	12,000	20,736

[1]Doctors without occupation including retired

Source: Author's summary from Bankowski and Fulop (1987), p. 20

Table 7.2 **World total of medical schools**

Year	Total	Number in developing countries	Percentage in developing countries
1955	646	241	37%
1960	756	336	45%
1970	1,004	493	49%
1975	1,151	591	51%
1983	1,344	739	55%

number of dentists required in the developed countries in the year 2015 will be about a quarter of those employed in 1985 (Bankowski and Fulop 1987: p. 26)[5]. Already dentists are unemployed or under-employed in Canada and Egypt.

International migration

In the past, surplus doctors were able to emigrate and often improved their economic prospects by doing so. In the 1950s and 1960s there was a large scale emigration of doctors from the Indian sub-continent to Britain while many British doctors who had failed to become specialists emigrated to Canada, Australasia and the United States (Gish 1971)[6]. For many years, the United States welcomed doctors from all over the world, provided that they could pass the ECFMG examination specially designed for emigrating doctors. By 1972, over half the candidates for state licensing examinations were foreign trained doctors (Stevens and Vermeulen 1972: p. ix)[7]. Indeed the medical curriculum in some medical schools in developing countries, such as the Philippines, became geared to enabling their graduates to pass this examination. Part of the reason for emigration was financial. But some emigrated because they could not find the type of work as a specialist for which they had been trained in their own country, or adequate facilities to do research (Abel-Smith and Gales 1964)[8]. A full 56 per cent of migrating doctors are from developing countries (World Bank 1993: box 6.1)[9].

These trends were criticised at the time for robbing the developing countries of doctors, trained usually at government expense, who were badly needed at home (UNTAR 1971, Stevens and Vermeulen 1972)[10]. It was seen as a vast subsidy from the developing world to the developed, not fully mitigated by the considerable financial remittances from these doctors to their families at home.

After the successive rises in the price of oil, starting in 1973, the newly rich Arab countries became doctor importers on a large scale. But from the 1980s, other countries became more restrictive in the admission of foreign medical graduates, partly due to pressure from their own graduates and partly due to political pressures to restrict the admission of every type of emigrant. Britain expanded its medical schools and planned to replace the foreign graduates, as they retired, with doctors trained at home. The United States also became more restrictive. This happened at the same time as reduced economic prospects made developing countries unable to employ all the doctors they had trained. Over the next two decades, the vast expansion of medical schools in the oil-rich Arab countries in the 1970s and 1980s will eventually enable them to replace foreigners with their own nationals. Thus many doctors who have practised high technological medicine in rich countries will find themselves sent back home.

The migration of doctors was followed by a migration of nurses which has been less well quantified. But the increase in nurses in the oil-exporting countries increased by 110 per cent between 1965 and 1980, largely owing to migration from India, Pakistan, the Philippines and Korea (Bankowski and Fulop 1987: p. 27)[11]. Nurses also move in large numbers from the Caribbean to the United States, leaving the country of origin with a shortage. In the 1980s, the United States addressed its nursing shortage by making it relatively easy for nurses to obtain visas. Jamaica was left with 50 per cent of unfilled vacancies and had to close whole wards as a result. About 90 per cent of migrating nurses go to North America, Europe and the high-income countries of the Western Pacific (World Bank 1993: box 6.1)[12].

Economic forces

Medicine is a field which has led to high earnings, at least for some doctors, in the past. And in many countries being a doctor led not only to a high income, but carried high prestige, was invulnerable to political instability and seemed to provide an international passport which was immune from confiscation. Economic theory would suggest that, when a profession becomes over-crowded, the income which can be earned from it is bound to fall and this would act as a signal to prospective entrants to choose another university course from which the economic prospects are brighter. But the market for doctors has many imperfections. First, in many countries there are strong medical trade unions which are able to maintain the salaries of doctors in employment, even though there are many young doctors who would willingly accept their jobs at a much lower salary. When salaries do fall in real terms, as they have in many African countries, this applies to the whole public sector of employment, and not to doctors alone. Similarly, the level of fees does not readily drop when there is a surplus of doctors, particularly when fees are negotiated under health insurance. Even in a private market where fees are not negotiated, the medical association tries to police any tendency to fee-cutting among their members. Second, where doctors are paid under health insurance on a fee-for-service basis, more and more doctors can be absorbed by over-servicing patients. Third, the most successful doctors may decide to take more leisure (for example, to play golf) and work only four days, thus releasing work for other doctors. Others may decide to retire early to enjoy their high savings.

Even if average earnings are falling and medical unemployment growing, this does not necessarily deter young people from entering the profession. Some may hope to emigrate, despite the falling opportunities. Prospective medical students who have a parent who is a doctor with a well-established practice may expect to start their clinical work by assisting their parent and eventually inherit the goodwill of the practice. Or a prospective student with the financial backing to be able to train as a specialist, particularly abroad, after the basic qualification, may expect to steal patients from local doctors without specialist qualifications. This feature is most noticeable in a country like Syria where central Damascus is festooned with doctors' signs advertising their qualifications and where they were obtained. The fact that average earnings are falling may not be inconsistent with continued very high earnings received by a minority of the most prestigious doctors. A prospective student is more likely to judge the financial prospects, not by the average, but by the continued availability of these glittering prizes. Finally, if medical unemployment does have some effect on deterring new entrants, this is bound to operate very slowly, simply because of the length of time it takes to be qualified as a doctor, let alone as a specialist.

Political pressures

In most countries the control, or at least the financing, of medical education is the responsibility of ministers of education, not health. The constituency lobbying the minister consists of parents ambitious for the educational opportunities of their children. In many Latin American countries, as in some European countries such as France, the right of any qualified student to select any university course has long been accepted and in some cases, following student revolutionary activity many years earlier, has been written into the constitution. The result is that medical courses become seriously over-crowded with the inevitable drop in standards. Ministers of education then come under pressure both from medical faculties and parents to relieve the pressure by opening new medical schools.

There are further political pressures for establishing more medical schools. If some provinces, or states, have medical schools, the others stake a claim for equal treatment. The demand comes from two sources. The first is parents wanting local educational opportunities for their children. The second is the local demand for the tertiary hospital which is normally associated with a medical school. This demand may come from a coalition of interests – doctors hoping for more senior appointments, local politicians with an eye on the job opportunities which will help to relieve local unemployment, and patients complaining about the absence locally of certain highly specialised medical facilities. Finally, it should not be overlooked that there must be few governments in the Third World without at least one minister with a son, daughter, niece or nephew hoping to enter medicine. In view of these political pressures, the case for more medical schools is likely to prevail even if the minister of health is concerned that further finance for tertiary hospitals will make it increasingly difficult to implement the priority for primary health care.

Professional prestige

Prestige is attached to practising specialised medicine in the United States and other developed countries. This is, moreover, the type of medical practice which the social and economic elite of developing countries expect to be able to find in their own country. In terms of financial rewards, doctors who can practise it expect to, and normally do, earn much more than those practising general medicine, let alone public health. Specialised surgery is normally the best rewarded and doctors who have trained in developed countries expect to earn more than those who have not, if they go back to developing countries.

These are powerful influences on the curricula of medical schools of developing countries. Some gear their curriculum to become what amounts to medical preparatory schools for specialist training abroad – even, in some cases, modelling it on the ECFMG examination to enter the United States. At the very least medical teachers in Third World countries want the qualifications they bestow to be recognised abroad – by the United Kingdom in many ex-British colonies and in France by many Francophone countries. As a result, it is still the case that external examiners travel to countries in Africa and Asia to validate their examinations.

The result of all these pressures is that the curriculum of medical schools in many developing countries is geared to the expectations of developed countries and the demands of the elite in the developing world, rather than to the needs of the major part of the local population. Thus doctors expect to have the support of sophisticated equipment in diagnosis and treatment wherever they work and their concern is with the disease pattern of the developed world rather than with the problems of malnutrition, diarrhoea and infectious disease which are the main problems facing the bulk of the developing world. Inevitably such doctors will not welcome an appointment to an under-equipped rural area where their main task will be to combat those health problems and give leadership to a team with a strong preventive orientation. They will not be willing to abandon the city life to which they have become accustomed at medical school, if they were not already accustomed to it before, for work in a rural area without electricity, safe water and good schools. Instead of doctors being trained in the situation and with the health problems where their work will be most needed, they have become ill-adapted both educationally and socially to coping with them. All this underlies the problem found far too often in developing countries of under-employed or unemployed doctors in urban areas while posts remain unfilled in rural areas.

Attracting and holding doctors for work in unpopular areas

Flooding the market with doctors does not necessarily solve the problem of geographical inequality. An excess of doctors will not necessarily lead to doctors settling in under-provided rural communities and slum neighbourhoods. This is true in both developed and developing countries. In so far as the doctor surplus does influence geographical inequality, the effect is bound to be uneven and will only happen after gross and costly over-provision in the popular areas.

The remedy of requiring a period of rural service in return for the medical education provided is less than satisfactory. Communities are faced with regular changes of doctor, few of whom have any roots in the community. Often their eye is on obtaining training as a specialist as soon as the period of rural service is over. This does not encourage them to acquire a deeper knowledge of the health problems of the communities where they are working or to develop long-term solutions to them. If a scholarship for specialist training has been promised after a satisfactory period of rural service, as is the practice in some countries (e.g. Chile), the long-term result is bound to be too many specialists and not enough generalists.

Some countries are attempting to remedy this by creating specialist qualifications in general practice with higher pay. This policy has been relatively successful in the United Kingdom. But it is difficult to establish it on a sufficient scale in developing countries, where doctors are allowed private practice after normal working hours and the remuneration for it greatly exceeds their government salary.

Attempts can be made to make rural postings more attractive by providing good housing with water and electricity at a very low rent, by providing a car (which can be retained after, for example, five years of rural service) and substantial extra allowances. Extra long leave can be given to those working in unpopular rural areas with their posts filled temporarily by other doctors, and allowances can be given to enable their children to attend boarding schools, if the standard of local schools is not acceptable. Assurances can be given that the longer a doctor works in a designated rural post, the more attractive the next post will be. 'The employer has a responsibility to develop a structure, climate and management style that will promote communication and make the best use of the skill and capacities of all those employed' (Simmonds and Bennet-Jones 1989: p. 3)[13]. But in some countries such measures would not provide a complete answer to this problem, at least to the extent that these extra provisions would be acceptable. The problem could be approached at the other end by requiring doctors in urban areas to pay a very high annual licensing fee to allow them to engage in private practice in urban areas, but such a logical solution is unlikely to win political support.

A more revolutionary approach is deliberately to recruit medical students from rural areas, even if their educational standard is lower, and establish a medical school in a rural area with a curriculum geared to the health needs of the local population, making use of district hospitals for most of the clinical experience. This would produce a different sort of doctor but one who had been trained from the start to work with health teams and focus on prevention rather than cure. Moreover, the cost of the medical education provided would be much lower.

The consequences of an excess of doctors

An excess of doctors is bound to be wasteful for a number of reasons. First, medical education is very expensive though it is hard to measure because of the difficulty of dividing up the costs of a teaching hospital (Abel-Smith *et al.* 1972)[14]. The cost per student in some developing countries was found in a study some years ago to be higher than in the United States or Britain (Abel-Smith *et al.* 1972)[15]. For the cost of training one doctor, several paramedicals could be trained. One developing country in which an attempt has been made to measure training costs is Pakistan, where it was estimated that for the cost of training one doctor, 2.5 nurses or six paramedicals could be trained (Abel-Smith 1987: p. 51)[16]. In East Africa, for the cost of training one doctor, two and a half nurses could be trained or 21 medical assistants (Bryant 1969: p. 123)[17].

Second, some doctors draw unemployment benefit. Others 'waste' their medical education, provided wholly or partly at government expense, by ending up in other occupations. Selling ice cream appears to be a common choice in Mexico and driving taxis in Argentina and Uruguay. Some go into business or take prestigious jobs in the public services or politics. It would be cheaper and more socially useful to allot more places in higher education to subjects offering a better preparation for these activities.

Third, unemployed doctors, particularly those whose families are well-connected politically, put pressure on governments to create urban jobs for doctors even when the highest priority is for more auxiliaries who are prepared to work in primary care in rural areas. More urban doctors add to costs much more than their salaries when allowance is made for the resources they need to support their work.

A fourth result may be over-servicing in the private sector, including the excessive use of expensive medical technology, thus raising unnecessarily the cost of medical care paid for by employers for their employees or by private citizens. Included in this over-servicing is a high use of drugs, which have a large import content, thus damaging the country's balance of payments.

It is not only developing countries which suffer the effects of an excess of medical personnel. Over-servicing is a well-established feature of the health care system in the United States, particularly in the use of diagnostic tests and surgery. Excessive use of diagnostic tests was also a feature of Belgium and Germany, until changes in the fee structure restrained further growth. In the European Community, where doctors have the right to work in any member state, the attempts of one country to plan its requirement for doctors are likely to be frustrated by immigration from other member states. All except two member states have placed limits on entry to medical school or raised the standard of the first year examinations. But most of these limits are designed to protect the standards of medical education rather than to restrict the long-term output of doctors to what the country can afford. There are still barriers of language, culture, post-graduate training and limits to entry to health insurance practice which limit this free movement, but these barriers are likely in the long run to be substantially reduced.

Planning the requirement for the health work-force

It is a fallacy to assume that the higher the ratio of doctors to population, the healthier the country will be. For example, there is no correlation between doctors per thousand population and the expectation of life among the developed countries. Nor is there a minimum ratio of doctors to population which a developing country 'needs' to have. Need is often a grossly misleading concept in health planning. What is relevant is not any theoretical need, however derived, but what a country can afford. This is true in developed countries as well as developing (Lapre 1973: pp. 111–23)[18]. Thus the relevant question is how many doctors will in the future be able to make a living in the public sector and the private sector combined, after allowing for any immigration and the absence of doctors gaining further training abroad. Within any total of expenditure for the public health sector, a balance must be kept between different grades of staff to ensure the accessibility of services. Inevitably, a poorer country will have to make greater use of paramedicals than a richer country, if all are to have access to services. Indeed the expected budget and the health plan should determine the exact balance. A method of doing this in primary care is presented in the next chapter.

Thus for each category of staff there needs to be an auxiliary grade. Such grades have different names in different countries. For example, those trained to diagnose and prescribe, within certain limitations, in Tanzania include not only assistant medical officers but medical assistants and rural medical aids. The latter only have primary education before their training programme.

This approach is often opposed on the argument that Third World countries ought to have the same quality of services as First World countries. It is said to be racialism or neocolonialism to argue that black people only need second rate 'doctors'. There are two answers to this criticism. First, there is no other way to provide services to all, unless fully trained doctors would be content with very low salaries. Second, it is restrictive practices, built up over the years, which have enabled the full professionals in developed countries to resist what they see as dilution. The evidence from developed countries is overwhelming that nurses with further training can be made fully competent to provide general practice. Indeed they do so under such titles as physician extenders in the United States. Similarly, dental assistants can provide a quality service of extractions and fillings under the supervision of a fully qualified dentist.

Much of what doctors do in developed countries could be done equally well or better by others. Is a doctor required to take a medical history, or could it be done by a nurse or medical secretary using a standard form? The doctor may wish to supplement it by some further pertinent questions. How much administrative work done by doctors could be delegated to others who could be trained to do it better? Should the instructions to relatives on the home care of the patient be given by a doctor or by a nurse who would provide that care if the patient were in hospital? The extent to which particular procedures are done by doctors or other staff depends on the customs of the country, the place of care, the remuneration system, legal provisions and fears of court cases for malpractice. Who provides anaesthetics, delivers babies, administers injections, takes out stitches and puts them in varies in different health care systems.

Routine procedures are not necessarily done better by persons with a lengthy professional education. Indeed the reverse may be the case. Where manual skill and conscientious attention to detail are required, the work may be better performed by those who do it frequently, are unrushed and are not distracted by considering other aspects of patient care. The nurse or paramedical worker, who takes blood specimens all day, will do a better job than the senior pathologist who only does it occasionally for private patients.

Training curricula

Each country should, therefore consider carefully what precise tasks persons with a university education are needed to perform, and design curricula accordingly. The same is true for those with a lower standard of education. For example, the main objective in Britain is not to try and teach medical students all that is known about medicine but to produce a doctor with 'a knowledge of the medical and behavioural sciences sufficient for him to go forward with medicine as it develops further' (*Royal Commission* 1968: p. 200)[19]. The mention of the behavioural sciences is important. There is some truth in the assertion that doctors study medicine which they do not practise and practise social sciences which they have not studied.

Many developing countries are training the wrong people for the wrong job. This contributes to the combination of unfilled vacancies in rural areas and unemployment in urban areas. In those developing countries where the majority of the population is rural, the functions of the doctors may be to plan, lead, supervise and train rather than undertake much medical work themselves. Training in management, supportive supervision, communication and team-work and inspirational leadership are all essential to the effectiveness and efficiency of health services. The doctor will need to know how to organise a sanitation campaign, arrange immunisation schedules, understand a growth curve and have a knowledge of local foods (Lechat and Borlee-Grimee 1987: pp. 509–10)[20]. Thus the doctor may need to know more about the job of other members of his or her rural health unit than about the work which is performed in the glossy teaching hospitals of the richer countries of the world. Moreover, those who are to work as a team should, in part, be taught together.

This does not mean that medical education will lack scientific rigour or make fewer intellectual demands. While the student may be spared the more sophisticated biochemistry, an expertise in epidemiology and statistics will be needed, as will the ability to examine alternative strategies and understand why particular priorities may be established from time to time. One of the glaring gaps in medical education is the lack of teaching of medical economics. A more relevant training leading to a qualification which need not be internationally recognised might not only improve performance but curb emigration. But medical schools are afraid to produce doctors who will not be recognised in the developed countries since they believe this would stamp them as inferior (Ransome-Kuti 1987: p. 163)[21].

Reform of this type is very difficult to achieve. A minister of health of Nigeria reports an attempt at reform at the University of Ife in his country. The original intention was not to build a large hospital but to use existing general hospitals and local health centres and dispensaries as a model for the national health system. Instead of appointing sociologists, public health doctors and general practitioners to build up primary care, the University appointed academics in the clinical and basic medical disciplines who changed the original philosophy and asked the Minister for a large teaching hospital. Another Nigerian University (Ilorin) did, however pioneer a relevant medical education. Its students were taught to identify health problems in the community and find solutions for them and were equipped with the skill to function in a hospital at an appropriate level in support of the community health services (Ransome-Kuti 1990: pp. 265–67)[22].

All over the world there is relative neglect of continuing education for all personnel working in the health sector. Only a few find the time and have the inclination to keep their practice up to date. Medical knowledge and techniques are continually expanding. The system of registration or licensing which confers the right to practise for life without further education or test of competence is increasingly being questioned. There is a growing demand for periodical further examinations to verify the competence of a doctor to continue in practice.

Planning the future health work-force

Once it is decided what staff can be afforded in the public sector in the long run, projections are needed on how many doctors are likely to be able to support themselves in the private sector. This requires up-to-date knowledge of existing personnel – their age, current deployment and presence in the country. This may need continuously updated computer records of each individual. (Wheeler and Ngcongco 1990: p. 394)[23]. This database can also be used to secure a rational distribution of current staff in relation to work load (Wheeler and Ngcongco 1990: p. 399)[24]. Crucial information, which many countries lack, is how many doctors are currently active in the private sector, to what extent retired doctors are still working and what tasks all these doctors are undertaking.

The next step is to plan to secure the right balance of health staff in the long run. The various steps needed to do this are shown in Table 7.3.

Table 7.3 **The process of planning the production of health staff**

Step 1. List current stock by category

Step 2. Project future supply on present policies
- the output of current training programmes
- deduct losses from deaths, retirements and any emigration

Step 3. Project demand based on affordability
- allow for any returning emigrants

Step 4. Match supply against affordable demand

Step 5. Increase or decrease planned output
- by more or less training institutions
- by cutting or increasing enrolment
- by stiffer educational requirements for entry

Step 6. Examine some key constraints
- calculate increase or decrease in the training budget required and feed back into estimated 'overhead' costs above
- consider willingness to work in rural areas
- consider the male/female balance according to the culture

The steps are simple and obvious. Start with a list of present staff by category. Calculate the likely available staff in the future if present policies are unchanged and compare this with the planned staff on the basis of affordability. Finally adjust the training policies so that the planned balance of staff will be available in the future. To implement such a policy may well involve painful political decisions. Closing a medical school is by no means easy: combining two schools is less contentious but the economies are lower. The least painful way forward politically is to reduce entry to all schools, but at some point this becomes grossly uneconomic.

All this may sound too idealistic and politically impossible. The United Kingdom has operated a policy of this kind for doctors with considerable success for the past 30 years, but this was when expansion was required. Contraction is much more difficult but has been particularly successfully managed by France even though quotas on entry to medical schools would be unacceptable. Raising the standard of the first year examinations is going a long way to achieve the desired result.

Conclusion

Planning the health professions, the mix of different grades, and where those who have been trained will practise are all critical for health service planning. If this is all left to market forces, any health system will become inequitable, unnecessarily expensive and unresponsive to health priorities. Moreover, there are important international ramifications which can seriously damage the best intentions of national planners. The developed countries have a responsibility not to allow their own selfish needs to obstruct health progress in the developing world.

Notes

1 Bankowski, Z. and Fulop, T. (1987), *Health Manpower out of Balance*, CIOMS, Geneva.
2 Roemer, M.I. (1988), 'Judging doctor supply – market or health criteria', *World Health Forum*, vol. 9.
3 Roemer (1988), 'Judging doctor supply'.
4 Bankowski and Fulop (1987), *Health Manpower*.
5 Bankowski and Fulop (1987), *Health Manpower*.
6 Gish, O. (1971), *Doctor Migration and World Health*, Occasional Papers in Social Administration No. 43, Bell, London.
7 Stevens, R. and Vermeulen, J. (1972), *Foreign Trained Physicians and American Medicine*, Department of Health Education and Welfare, Washington D.C.
8 Abel-Smith, B. and Gales, K. (1964), *British Doctors at Home and Abroad*, Occasional Papers in Social Administration, No. 8, Bell, London.
9 World Bank (1993), *World Development Report 1993: Issues in Health*, World Bank, Washington D.C.
10 See UNTAR (1971), *The Brain Drain from Five Developing Countries, Research Reports*, NO. 5, UNTAR, New York, 1971; Stevens and Vermeulen (1972), *Foreign Trained Physicians*.
11 Bankowski and Fulop (1987), *Health Manpower*.
12 World Bank (1993), *World Development Report*.
13 Simmonds, S. and Bennet-Jones, N. (1989), *Human Resource*

Development: The Management, Planning and Training of Health Personnel, EPC Publication No. 21, London School of Hygiene and Tropical Medicine.

14 Abel-Smith, B. *et al.* (1972), 'Can we reduce the costs of medical education?', *WHO Chronicle*, vol. 2, no. 10.

15 Abel-Smith *et al.* (1972), 'Can we reduce the costs'.

16 Abel-Smith, B. (1987), 'The cost of unbalanced manpower', in Bankowski and Fulop *Health Manpower*.

17 Bryant, J. (1969), *Health in the Developing World*, Cornell University Press, Ithaca.

18 Lapre, R.M. (1973), 'Planning of medical manpower for health care in the light of a changing employment market', in Jaspers, C.A., *Health Manpower Planning*, Martinus Nijhoff, The Hague.

19 *Royal Commission on Medical Education, 1965–6*, (1968), Cmnd. 3569, HMSO, London.

20 Lechat, M.F., and Borlee-Grimee, I. (1987), 'Training medical students to practise in the Third World', *World Health Forum*, vol. 8, no. 4.

21 Ransome-Kuti, O. (1987), 'Finding the right road to health', *World Health Forum*, vol. 8, no. 2.

22 Ransome-Kuti, O. (1990), 'A new breed of doctors', *World Health Forum*, vol. 11.

23 Wheeler, M. and Ngcongco, V.N. (1990), 'Health manpower planning in Botswana', *World Health Forum*, vol. 11.

24 Wheeler and Ngcongco (1990), 'Health manpower planning'.

CHAPTER 8

Planning primary health care

According to WHO's global strategy of 1981, 'primary health care is the key to obtaining health for all' (WHO 1989)[1].

It is essential care made universally accessible to individuals and families in the community by means acceptable to them, through their full participation and at a cost the community and country can afford. It forms an integral part both of the country's health systems of which it is the nucleus and the overall social and economic development of the country. (WHO 1978: p. 2)[2]

Why primary care was given priority

The emphasis on primary health care originated in five underlying ideas. The first was a recognition of the importance of inter-sectoral action for health development. This grew out of the discussion of development from the middle 1960s, which recognised that economic growth did not necessarily 'trickle down' to the poor, as economists had too readily assumed, and that the central problem of development was how to meet the basic needs of the poor. Economic and social development were not separate but closely inter-related.

The second reason was the recognition, based on experience of earlier programmes, that the key infectious diseases could not be successfully combated by specific isolated programmes of mass campaigns against particular diseases controlled from the centre. In the long run, it was not effective to have one 'vertical' programme aimed at water and sanitation, another at malaria, and a third at leprosy. This was because all programmes needed the support of local health staffs and local populations (Brockington 1985: p. 199)[3]. The most striking failure of WHO had been the malaria eradication programme on which it had staked and lost a considerable amount of its credibility. Substantial progress was achieved by centrally directed activity but mosquitoes developed in Darwinian fashion which were resistant to the chemicals that were used (Brockington 1985: p. 51)[4]. The lesson was not lost on Dr Mahler, who had controlled the malaria programme in India before he became Director-General of WHO and launched the 'Health for All' programme.

The third underlying idea was that preventive and promotive action should not be separated from curative action. This was the way in which services had developed in most countries, both developed and developing. Often, under the chief medical officer would be found a deputy for curative services and a deputy for preventive services. The origin of the separation was that prevention and promotion were seen as collective responsibilities while curative action, except in the case of the major infectious diseases, was an individual responsibility. Moreover, clinicians in most countries had developed as self-employed professionals, paid by patients, and later their insurers, while preventive action had always required doctors paid salaries and employed by government. The division of the profession was reflected in the division of services.

The development of compulsory health insurance crystallised the separation in most countries. This was because the precise boundary of what was and what was not covered by health insurance had to be defined. As preventive services were already being provided by government, they were not brought within the original scope of health insurance. The definition became sharpest when doctors insisted on being paid on a fee-for-service basis as in Germany and France. The 'medical acts' for which fees were payable to doctors did not include preventive services.

Fourth was the evidence that there was a range of health activities which were relatively cheap and very effective which nevertheless did not reach millions of people throughout the world.

The improvement of health is being equated with the provision of medical care dispensed by growing numbers of specialists, using narrow medical technologies for the benefit of the privileged few . . . The concentration of complex and costly technology on limited segments of the population does not even have the advantage of improving health. (Brockington 1985: p. 7)[5].

Finally, it represented a strong reaction against authoritarian attempts of the health professions to impose health on people.

Self reliance and social awareness are key factors in human development . . . [Community participation] enables them to become agents of their own development instead of beneficiaries of development aid . . . Of overriding importance is the principle that public services should be accountable to the communities they serve, in particular for resources that the latter have invested. (Brockington 1985: pp. 19–20)[6].

The content of primary care

The next step after 'Health for All' was endorsed in 1977, was to sponsor a world conference to secure agreement on the content of primary health care as shown in Table 8.1. This conference was held in Alma Ata in the former Soviet Union, the only country prepared at the time to give the financial backing needed for the conference.

The new policy emphasised equity, a focus on prevention, inter-sectoral action, community participation, and appropriate technology.

Table 8.1   **The elements of primary care**

---

1. PROMOTION of proper nutrition and an adequate supply of safe water;

2. Basic SANITATION;

3. MATERNAL AND CHILD HEALTH CARE including family planning;

4. IMMUNISATION against the major infectious diseases;

5. PREVENTION and control of locally endemic diseases;

6. EDUCATION concerning prevailing health problems and the methods of preventing and controlling them;

7. Appropriate TREATMENT of common diseases and injuries;

8. Provision of essential DRUGS.

The first four chapters stressed the importance of inter-sectoral action. There is room for disagreement on the meaning of equity, appropriate technology and community involvement.

Equity

The Alma Ata conference urged that priority should be given to those who are least able for geographical, political, social or financial reasons to take the initiative in seeking health care. Those most vulnerable or at greatest risk were women, children, working populations at high risk and the underprivileged segments of society.

The aim is that health resources should be equitably distributed. This is of critical importance for primary health care. Moreover, equity can be achieved quicker in the case of primary health care than in hospitals which, once built, cannot readily be moved. Equity in health services can provide some compensation for inequalities elsewhere in the society, and health services can bring tangible benefits to rural populations which cannot as rapidly be achieved in other sectors.

Equity can have many meanings. First, it is intended to mean geographical equity. Second, it means financial accessibility: people are not deterred by money barriers. Third, it includes cultural accessibility: the technical and managerial methods used are in keeping with the cultural patterns of the community. Fourth, it means functional accessibility: the right kind of care is available on a continuing basis to those who need it, whenever they need it (Brockington 1985: p. 29)[7].

At first sight, it may seem that equity is achieved if health resources are distributed geographically equally per head of the population to be served. The population served is not the same as the population resident, as some of the latter may insist on using private sector services and others go long distances to obtain what they think will be better care. But such a formula would take no account of health need. An alternative formulation of equity would be equal provision for equal need. Thus areas with greater health needs would be given more resources to try to meet these extra needs. But this takes no account of the cost of meeting need in different areas. It will be more expensive to make services accessible to dispersed populations: health units may have to have low utilisation and therefore be more expensive and more transport may be needed for referral and supervision.

But accessibility does not solve the whole problem. The poor and poorly educated may not present their needs. In some countries health professionals are less welcoming to them and make the lower income groups feel inferior by 'talking down to them'. This problem can to some extent be reduced by training. But much depends on the financial incentives facing the health professional. If extra patients lead to extra money for the staff, they are likely to be more welcoming to all patients, just as with a shop-keeper. Those who ought to attend but do not are an important potential source of extra income. But services may need to be taken to very small communities or even to homes. Extensive health education may be needed to get acceptance of the advantages of immunisation, antenatal care and family planning or to make people aware that not all conditions can be treated effectively by traditional practitioners.

An increasing number of developed countries are using different types of population-based formulas to distribute resources for health. This is the case in Italy (Abel-Smith 1984: p. 70)[8], New Zealand and the United Kingdom. In the United Kingdom a formula was used to distribute finance for the health services which took into account not only the age and sex of the population served but mortality rates as a proxy for morbidity (see, e.g. Le Grand *et al*. 1990: pp. 166–20)[9]. Any attempt to push health resources in favour of those with the greatest health needs will challenge the expectations of the more vocal urban section of the population. A government which shifts the balance in favour of the relatively deprived majority is also shifting the basis of its support, but the new power base may prove more stable than the old one in the long run.

One developing country which does succeed in favouring the poorer areas is Costa Rica. In the poorest region of the country, 37 per cent more per head is spent on health services than in the richest region (Abel-Smith and Creese 1989: p. 142)[10]. Those identified as poor are 6 per cent of the population but they use about one third of all health resources (Abel-Smith and Creese 1989: p. 135)[11]. Inevitably the poor include many chronically sick and aged persons.

Appropriate technology

'Appropriate technology means that, besides being scientifically sound, the technology is also acceptable to those who apply it and to those for whom it is applied. This means that technology should be in keeping with the local culture' (WHO 1978: p. 29)[12]. 'It also means treating people in their situation (urban conurbation or small village) in the least-cost and most effective way consistent with the severity of the problem' (Lee 1985: p. 103)[13].

Community participation

The Alma Ata declaration placed great emphasis on community involvement. 'Community participation is the process by which individuals and families assume responsibility for their own health and welfare and for those of the community, and develop the capacity to contribute to their own and their community's development' (WHO 1978: p. 20)[14]. The inclusion of the word 'welfare' is critical. It implies that health should be defined in the context of better living conditions, including housing, agriculture and employment opportunities. The community 'must first be involved in the assessment of the situation, the definition of problems and the setting of priorities' (WHO 1978: p. 21)[15]. This implies a 'bottom up' approach to health planning. Then the community should keep the implementation of primary health care under constant review and make sure that it functions in accordance with its stated purpose (WHO 1978: p. 21)[16].

There can, however, be different degrees of involvement:

- Collaboration implies shared decision-making by equal partners with overlapping responsibilities;
- Participation implies collaboration without all participating groups having responsibility for the area of interest;
- Consultation is the seeking of advice and opinion without a commitment to follow the views received;
- Negotiation is where one body cannot get what it wants without seeking accommodation with another party (Lee and Mills 1982: p. 129)[17].

The case for involvement has been argued as a means simply of extending democracy, to improve the quality of decisions or to redress the power of government or the professions. It is argued that the community should be involved not just in the planning of local services but in their administration. 'Involvement of the people is not only a way to get things done, but also to increase understanding, maintain interest and develop self-reliance: it lessens the resistance to change' (Brockington 1985: p. 196)[18].

One way forward is the appointment of committees representative of the community to work with primary health care teams. Inevitably this involves a transfer of power from health professionals to local laypeople and this challenges the traditional thinking, and often training, of those professionals who have come to believe that they always know best. The challenge is greatest where health professionals have fought for and won a wide degree of autonomy and are working in independent competitive practice. Local participation challenges deep-rooted attitudes – particularly in many developed countries. It takes time for attitudes to change, and the imposition of alien ideas can be counterproductive in its effect as a number of experiences have shown. Change is likely to come, not through direction from above, but through example from below.

A study has shown just how difficult it is for these aims to be achieved (Rifkin 1985)[19]. Some accept the approach intellectually but act in a technical way. Community members often failed to see health as a high priority compared with housing, food production or income generation. Often there has been a failure to recognise the diversity of communities, their power groups and basic inequalities.

Affordable services

WHO made it clear that its aim was not to expand primary health care at the expense of other services when the 12 world health indicators were agreed in 1981. One of the indicators was that expenditure on health services should, by the year 2000, amount to at least 5 per cent of each country's gross domestic product – a figure well ahead of what most developing countries were spending. It was assumed tacitly that world economic growth would continue to increase on the same scale and that countries would be able to find more money for the national health budget (WHO 1978: p. 12)[20]. It was also hoped foreign donors would increase their assistance to the developing countries' health efforts, now that clear aims and priorities had been articulated (WHO 1978: p. 47)[21]. All these hopes were shattered by the economic crisis described in chapter 11.

In practice, affordability led to considerable reliance being placed on community health workers. They are

local people who are not expected to move away from the communities they serve. They are preferably women, but some programmes are dominated by men. They receive a very short training, and unlike other health professionals, they are unlikely to have the opportunity to be promoted to higher positions, or to be transferred to another part of the country. In most programmes they are generally paid a salary or honorarium and are identified closely with the health service. For the most part they act as extenders of health services rather than as development or change agents. (Walt 1988: p. 4)[22].

The use of community health workers has not been without its problems, particularly in their relationships with nurses (Walt 1988: p. 1–21)[23]. It has been difficult to persuade medically unqualified people that they are capable of giving services, and to convince communities to accept them. Often community members who participated expected planners to provide the services while the planners expected the community members to provide the health care. And where this was the case, the cost to them was not fully appreciated in terms of the money and opportunities sacrificed.

Decentralisation

The policy envisaged substantial decentralisation of services to provincial and district levels. 'These levels are near enough to respond sensitively to their practical problems and needs: they are equally near to the central administrative level to translate government policies into practice' (Walt 1988: p. 22)[24]. Decentralisation can have many meanings. A distinction is often made between deconcentration (handing powers over to local offices of the ministry), devolution (handing powers over to local government) and delegation (handing over defined functions to, for example, local boards or parastatals) (Rondinelli 1981: pp. 133–34)[25].

In deciding between different forms, the questions to be answered are what is to be decentralised to whom and why. The purposes may be, for example, to encourage inter-sectoral action, to create community participation, or to move decision-makers nearer to the services, so that they are better informed and the services better coordinated, to speed decision-making or to release the time of those at the top from questions of detail for strategic thinking, supportive supervision or continuing education for staff. If the purpose is just to take the load off the top, then delegation or deconcentration are a means of doing this. If the main aim is inter-sectoral coordination then powers can be devolved to elected local government or governors responsible to a co-ordinating central government department (local government, the interior or the president's office). The powers handed over may be legislative, revenue-raising, policy-making, resource allocation, the deployment of the work-force, regulation, management, inter-sectoral collaboration, and/or training. If the main aim is community participation, substantial powers need to be given to the district level or below. Often more than one of these purposes underlies the drive towards decentralisation. A major issue is the competence of local authorities to take responsibility for health in view of their weak tax base.

Decentralisation is by no means easy. For this reason there are advantages in gradually phasing it in. The precise functions transferred must be clearly defined and there will be constant pressures to reduce or stretch them. It will take time for those to whom powers are handed to be trained to use them and gain practice in doing so. Similarly, a major adjustment of roles is needed at the centre. The process requires continuous development and adaptation.

Team-working

WHO envisages that the professionals working in primary health care will not just apply their separate skills to contribute to the care of individual patients but work together as a team to find ways of improving the health of the community. In the past, the essence of primary care was continuity of relationships so that knowledge was acquired of each patient's medical history, family setting and ideally also his or her occupational setting, all of which may be relevant to the care of the patient's health. The new approach adds the dimension of the community. What are the reasons for differences in health of different social groups? What features of the local environment, diet and culture are favourable or unfavourable to health? What aspects of behaviour are health-damaging? What are local health practices and where else are health advice and care obtained? What is the best way of attempting to initiate change? 'Primary health care cannot be isolated or treated apart from the complexities of beliefs and customs: at almost every turn it involves adjustments, some fundamental in the cultural framework' (Brockington 1985: p. 191)[26]. Thus the primary health team members will hold regular meetings to compare notes in making a community diagnosis and plan their collective activities in discussion with the local community.

Selecting an affordable labour mix

WHO envisaged that primary health care would mobilise the human potential of the entire community (WHO 1978: p. 31)[27]. At the first level of contact between individuals and the health care system there were to be community health workers who would act as a team. The types of health worker would vary according to needs and the resources for satisfying them. They could vary from people with very limited education but with an elementary training in health care, as mentioned above, to medical assistants, practical or professional nurses, general practitioners or traditional practitioners (WHO 1978: pp. 31–32)[28]. For developing countries it was envisaged that community health workers would be trained in a short time to perform specific tasks.

The first step is to work out what work-force can be afforded out of a given health budget which is expected to be available to be spent on primary health care in the long run – ten or fifteen years ahead. Out of this budget, sums would need to be put aside for overheads – tertiary and specialised hospitals, training and central administrative functions (including central laboratories, and stores). The remaining budget, which is available for primary health care, is then divided into population groups of 100,000. A proportion (based largely on current experience) is set aside for supplies – say 40 per cent. This leaves 200,000 currency units to be spent on staff per 100,000 population. Possible ways of using these 200,000 currency units are shown in Table 8.2.

Table 8.2 **Staffing options for spending 200,000 currency units per 100,000 population**

Grade by level of education	Annual salary	Number in post options		
		A	B	C
UNIVERSITY	20,000	10	6	2
SECONDARY + 3 YEARS TRAINING	6,000	0	10	10
PRIMARY + 6 MONTHS TRAINING	2,000	0	10	50

N.B. The total salary cost for each option adds up to 200,000 currency units.

To simplify the example, it is assumed that there are only three grades of staff – those with a university education, those with secondary education and further training of two or three years and those with a primary education followed by training for six months. More grades of staff can be fitted into the same type of table.

In this example the first option (A) is for ten university-trained staff (doctors, dentists or pharmacists) per 100,000 population without any supporting staff. It is quite clear that it would be impossible to provide accessibility in rural areas with this option unless the whole population had access to motorised transport. Moreover it would be wasteful to deploy highly trained staff without any support, as they would have to undertake tasks which could readily be done by those with less training. The second option (B) provides six university-trained staff. Two or three of them might look after the district hospital, leaving the others to supervise and take referrals from less than perhaps six subsidiary health units, each with two staff, as the district hospital will need some supporting staff. It would not be possible to provide ready access on this basis. The third option (C) at least makes it possible to provide two staff of the lowest level of training in health units serving some 4,000 persons plus one more senior one in larger units, while leaving workers to staff and support the district hospital. Thus the choice of option depends on the importance attached to accessibility which will of course, vary between urban and rural areas. Once the tasks of the various staff have been sketched out, a check would need to be made on whether the allowance of 40 per cent of the budget for non-staff costs still seems appropriate.

The above over-simplified model does not allow for staff leave, sickness and refresher courses. Moreover at this stage it is appropriate also to reconsider the original allocation for overheads. Is it possible to spend less on tertiary hospitals and specialised hospitals so as to increase spending on primary care? Are tertiary hospitals being used as they are intended to be used – only for patients referred from lower levels of the health care system, because it is only at the tertiary hospitals that the facilities are available to treat them? As will be discussed in chapter 10, this is very often not the case. If steps can be phased in to correct this over the years, more can be allocated to primary health care and the options in the above table can be made more expensive. Once the work-force mix has been decided, the second step is to allocate this work-force and other resources between the areas of 100,000 population on an equitable basis.

Planning the services

The planning of services depends on the density of population. In an urban area, services can be based on health centres. In rural areas with limited motorised transport, there may need to be health centres and beneath them dispensaries or health posts with perhaps only two paid staff, one concentrating mainly on curative work and immunisation, and the other mainly on maternal and child health with help from community health workers. Where population is very dispersed, the health centre may have to have similar staffing to a dispensary, with the addition of a more senior health worker to supervise the outlying services. The district hospital may be at the health centre or serving several health centres. Where transport is of limited availability, all units may need one or more beds for holding seriously ill patients until they can be taken to the hospital, as well as beds for delivery.

Selective primary health care

By 1980, there were some who were arguing that the very broad concept of primary health care agreed at Alma Ata was too ambitious and expensive. Would a narrower definition be more realistic? It was argued that the need was to institute 'selective primary health care directed at preventing or treating those few diseases responsible for the greatest mortality in less developed areas and for which interventions of proven high efficacy exist' (Walsh and Warren 1980: p. 145)[29]. What was proposed was immunisation for children (measles and DPT) and pregnant mothers (tetanus), long-term breast feeding, chloroquine for children under three, and oral rehydration.

Essentially this was a return to the CENDES approach discussed in chapter 6, but on a global scale. It was attractive to some donors because of the cost-effective argument and the measurable results (Unger and Killingworth 1986: p. 1001)[3]. It was criticised on ethical grounds for giving services only to children and mothers and its practicability was questioned. But much more fundamentally, it was attacked for seeing health only in disease terms, for ignoring equity, for not recognising the multi-sectoral approach to health and failing to see health 'as the result of the motivation, attitudes and action of individuals and communities who are slowly beginning to define their role and responsibility in health care' (Rifkin and Walt 1986: pp. 559–66)[31].

In 1987, as part of its advocacy of 'adjustment with a human face' (Cornia *et al.* 1987)[32], UNICEF argued that in the short term the well-being of vulnerable groups can be better protected by better resource allocation (targeting). This was the GOBI-FFF strategy (Growth monitoring, Oral rehydration therapy, Breast Feeding, Immunisation, Family spacing, Food supplements and Female Education). This policy can be attacked on much the same basis. 'Implicit in the GOBI-FFF strategy is the view that selective intervention can improve health, without the improvement in people's economic social and political environment. The strategy depoliticises health and naturalises poverty' (Kanji 1989: p. 113)[33]. Several of the interventions proposed have considerable limitations. Growth monitoring is costly in time and effort if accurate data is to be obtained (Henri *et al* 1989: pp. 395–400)[34], oral dehydration does not help all forms of diarrhoea (Feacham 1986: pp. 109–17)[35] and it is difficult to influence family spacing. The strategy seemed attractive to some donors because at least immunisation and oral rehydration could give short-term results which can be quantified.

The reception of primary care in developing countries

The reception of the primary care approach in developing countries has been variable. Some countries have seen it as only a second-class service for marginal populations lacking access to hospitals (Cabral 1990: p. 435)[36]. There has also been some failure to appreciate that the eight essential elements could not all be covered at the first contact level and that the technical, training and management support of a hospital at the first level is essential (Dujardin 1989: p. 430)[37]. But other countries, provided they had sufficient resources, have tried to make a success of the approach. Still others (particularly in Africa) have become increasingly short of resources to do so. Increasingly they have become reliant on donors to keep their services going. In some countries different donors have taken responsibility for different sections of the programme or for different regions. In some cases national structures and institutions have been bypassed or weakened through donor intervention. In the attempt to achieve targets, the expanded programme of immunisation has often been carried out by 'top down' mass campaigns with measurable results, giving the mistaken impression that health is something which comes from the capital in four-wheel drives. On the other hand immunisation coverage has shot ahead from 5 per cent of the world's children immunised against the six target diseases in 1977 to 50 per cent in 1987. But there is evidence that community participation is needed to achieve very high rates (Kowli *et al* 1990: pp. 169–72)[38]. Similarly, there has been a tendency for donors to develop 'top down' vertical programmes for essential drugs, family planning and AIDS – each with its own separate educational component. Such programmes do not develop long-term capacity or transfer knowledge, information or skills let alone empowerment. The lack of coordination and duplication can result in the non-sustainability of these donor-run vertical programmes (Bossert 1990: pp. 1019–20)[39].

The reception of primary care in the developed countries

By 1978, when the Alma Ata declaration was promulgated, a number of developed countries were already giving priority to primary health care and were bringing together their preventive and curative services where these had developed separately. A bridge between preventive and curative care had been forged in the United Kingdom partly by offering fees to general practitioners for defined preventive work and partly by attaching health visitors and, to a lesser extent midwives to general practices with their salaries separately paid through the National Health Service. In Sweden and Finland, integrated primary health units had been developed with salaried doctors. To these countries, integrated primary health care represented less of a challenge. But full integration was less acceptable in continental Europe.

In 1982, the Director of the European Region of WHO presented draft targets to the regional committee which is constituted by the ministries of health of the region. The priority to be given to primary health care did not create dissension. It could be presented as a means of containing costs which fitted with most of the countries' current concerns. But the draft included a very comprehensive concept of primary health care as shown in Table 8.3. The items which greatly extended the traditional concept of primary health care are shown in italics.

This concept was not acceptable to many of the European countries. First, it implied a major reorientation of the medical education system towards prevention and health promotion. Second, and most important, it suggested that medical care given by doctors working alone from their own offices or even in groups would have to give way to teams of health professionals. The type of team work envisaged does not fit with traditional education and training of health professionals which was aimed at imparting the relevant separate skills, not at collaboration in joint efforts of this kind.

A delicate point is who should lead the team. In the long run, would it be a specialist in public health or even a social worker rather than a doctor whose skills and experience lay in curative medicine? To

Table 8.3   **Draft European targets for primary health care, 1982**

1. COVERAGE OF PREVENTION, PROMOTION AND CURE
   - Family Planning *including genetic counselling,*
   - Home care including nursing,
   - Immunisation and selective screening,
   - *Integrated* maternal and child health,
   - *Occupational and school health,*
   - *Rehabilitation,*
   - *Counselling on lifestyle,*
   - *Education and self-care,*
   - *Links with ALL self-help groups,*
   - *Epidemiological surveillance of disease.*

2.   *BASED ON COMMUNITY PARTICIPATION*

3.   PROVIDING 24 HOUR EMERGENCY *SERVICE*

4.   REACH OUT INTO HOMES, *SCHOOLS AND JOBS*

5.   TEAM TO INCLUDE:

Doctor	*Physiotherapist*	*Pharmacist*
Nurse	*Social worker*	*Sanitarian*
Midwife	*Dentist*	*Possibly*
		Health educator

suggest that it may not always be a clinical doctor is to challenge existing assumptions of authority and responsibility. This was a particularly sensitive issue in countries where doctors were paid on a fee-for-service system under health insurance. Other members of the team would assume tasks, some of which were covered by the fee schedule only payable to doctors. Were salaries to be substituted for other ways of paying primary care doctors? Governments were lobbied by medical interests, particularly in Belgium, France and Germany. As a result, the Regional Office of WHO had to come back with a much more anodyne draft which was endorsed two years later. This does not mean that no progress was made. For example, during the 1980s both Spain and Portugal took steps to bring together their preventive and curative primary services on the same premises.

Conclusion

The thrust to primary health care will not happen without strong political support. This is true of both developed and developing countries. It is likely to encounter opposition both from leading clinicians and from the more affluent and vocal section of the population who want direct access to what they consider the best qualified doctors. Where this direct access has become the norm, the health care system becomes unaffordable even for the richest countries. Thus the primary health initiative is of critical relevance to countries at all levels of development.

Notes

1   World Health Organisation (1989), *Formulating Strategies for Health For All by the Year 2000*, WHO, Geneva.
2   World Health Organisation (1978), *Primary Health Care*, WHO, Geneva.
3   Brockington, F. (1985), *The Health of the Developing World*, Book Guild, Lewes.
4   Brockington (1985), *Health of the Developing World*.
5   Brockington (1985), *Health of the Developing World*.
6   Brockington (1985), *Health of the Developing World*.
7   Brockington (1985), *Health of the Developing World*.
8   Abel-Smith, B., (1984), *Cost Containment in Health Care*, Bedford Square Press, London.
9   Le Grand, J., *et al.* (1990), 'The National Health Service: safe in whose hands', in Hills, J. (ed.) *The State of Welfare*, Oxford.
10 Abel-Smith, B. and Creese, A. (1989), *Recurrent Costs in the Health Sector*, WHO, Geneva.
11 Abel-Smith and Creese (1989), *Recurrent Costs*.
12 WHO (1978), *Primary Health Care*.
13 Lee, K. (1985), 'Resources and costs in primary health care' in Lee, K. and Mills, A. (eds.), *The Economics of Health in Developing Countries*, Oxford.
14 WHO (1978), *Primary Health Care*.
15 WHO (1978), *Primary Health Care*.
16 WHO (1978), *Primary Health Care*.
17 Lee, K. and Mills, A. (1982), *Policy-making and Planning in the Health Sector*, Croom Helm.
18 Brockington (1985), *Health of the Developing World*.
19 Rifkin, S.B. (1985), *Health Planning and Community Participation*, Beckenham.
20 WHO (1978), *Primary Health Care*.
21 WHO (1978), *Primary Health Care*.
22 Walt, G. (1988), 'CHWs: are the national programmes in crisis?', *Health Planning and Policy*, vol. 3, no. 1.
23 Walt (1988), 'CHWs'.
24 Walt (1988), 'CHWs'.
25 Rondinelli, D.A. (1981), 'Government decentralisation in comparataive Perspective: theory and practice in developing countries' *International Review of Administrative Science*, vol. 47, no, 2.
26 Brockington (1985), *Health of the Developing World*.
27 WHO (1978), *Primary Health Care*.
28 WHO (1978), *Primary Health Care*.
29 Walsh, L.A. and Warren, K.E. (1980), 'Selective primary health care: an interim strategy for disease control in developing countries'. *Social Science and Medicine*, vol. 14c.

30   Unger, J.P. and Killingworth, J. (1986), 'Selective primary health care: a critical review of methods and results', *Social Science and Medicine*, vol. 20.

31   Rifkin, S.B. and Walt, G. (1986), 'Why health improves: defining the issues concerning comprehensive primary care and selective primary care, *Social Science and Medicine*, vol. 23.

32   Cornia, G. *et al.* (1987), *Adjustment with a Human Face*, Clarendon, Oxford.

33   Kanji, N. (1989), 'Charging for drugs in Africa', *Health Policy and Planning*, vol. 4, no. 2.

34   Henri, F. *et al.* (1989), 'Targeting nutritional interventions: is there a role for growth monitoring', *Health Policy and Planning*, vol. 4, no. 4.

35   Feacham, R.G. (1986), 'Preventing diarrhoea: what are the policy options?, *Health Policy and Planning*, vol. 1, no. 2.

36   Cabral, A.J.R. (1990), 'Maintaining the health-for-all momentum', *World Health Forum*, vol. 11.

37   Dujardin, B. (1989), 'Hospitals for primary health care', *World Health Forum*, vol. 10.

38   Kowli, S.K. *et al.* (1990), 'Community participation boosts immunisation coverage', *World Health Forum*, vol. 11.

39   Bossert, T.J., (1990), 'Can they get along without us? Sustainability of donor-supported health projects in Central America and Africa, *Social Science and Medicine*, vol. 30, no. 9.

CHAPTER 9

Planning pharmaceuticals

Expenditure on pharmaceuticals normally amounts to 10 to 20 per cent of health expenditure in developed countries and 20 to as much as 60 per cent of expenditure in developing countries. The proportion of expenditure tends to be higher in developing countries than in developed, because labour costs are lower in the former, and at least the basic ingredients, if not the finished products, have normally to be imported and prices are set internationally. From a health point of view, the purpose of planning pharmaceutical expenditure is to secure value for money. This means that the drugs purchased need to be safe, effective, rationally prescribed and distributed without waste to where they are needed. Countries with balance of payment problems have a special interest in ensuring that drugs are used economically in view of their high import content.

Prescribing

The most commonly used medicines throughout the world are those taken without a prescription. This is true in both developed and developing countries. Osler once remarked that 'a desire to take medicines is perhaps the greatest feature which distinguishes man from other animals'[1]. The persons who most commonly decide what drugs should be taken are the patient and the family, not the doctor. For example a study found that only 16 per cent of reported symptoms in Britain are taken to the doctor (Herxheimer and Stimson 1981: p. 48)[2]. Every society has its ranges of what can be described as traditional medicines. In a developing country, these may be herbs bought in the market or preparations provided by the traditional doctor as part of treatment, as used to be the case in the United Kingdom before general practitioners separated from apothecaries. Japanese doctors still dispense the drugs they prescribe. In developed countries 'household remedies' are bought from supermarkets, pharmacists or drug stores. About 15 over-the-counter drugs per person per year are bought in Britain compared with 6.5 prescription drugs. Over half the population uses one each day (Herxheimer and Stimson 1981: p. 48)[3]. Household remedies are more used by women than men, smokers rather than non-smokers, whites rather than blacks and those with lower rather than higher prescribed drug costs (Blum and Kreitman 1981: p. 128)[4].

Studies have shown that both in Britain and the United States, the average household has in stock about 17 household remedies and 5 prescribed drugs (Herxheimer and Stimson 1981: p. 51, Blum and Kreitman 1981: p. 127)[5]. Two-thirds of the sales are for analgesics, digestives, laxatives, cough and cold remedies and vitamins (Herxheimer and Stimson 1981: p. 51)[6]. Over-the-counter drugs are heavily advertised: for example, one commercial slot in eight on American television was for a non-prescription drug.

Even in the case of prescription drugs, it is the patient, rather than the doctor, who decides what drugs are taken. One careful study in the United States showed that only 22 per cent of prescribed drugs are taken as directed, 30 per cent are misused in a way which posed a threat to health and 8 per cent of admissions to hospital were due to adverse drug reactions (Blum and Kreitman 1981: pp. 143, 151)[7]. While over-the-counter drugs are the most common drugs taken, prescribed drugs are on average much more expensive. Thus the waste of these drugs is a more important issue.

Prescribing is an important part of doctors' practices. Most patients get a prescription at the end of a consultation. Prescribing is part of the psychological relationship between doctor and patient. It also has latent functions. One is to validate the patient's visit – to reassure the patient that he or she was right to come to see the doctor. In many societies, patients who fail to receive a drug will interpret this as being told that they are not ill and the doctor often finds it safer to assume an illness than to deny it. Thus the prescription legitimises 'the sick role' in the family. If the patient is paying for the consultation, receiving a prescription is obtaining something tangible for the payment to the doctor. It satisfies the patient's expectations. It would take up more of the time of the doctor to explain why no drug was necessary: prescribing something is less time-consuming. And repeat prescriptions are a commitment to a continuing doctor–patient relationship. Prescribing also demonstrates the knowledge and power of the doctor. Finally, it enables the doctor politely to terminate the consultation. This can pose difficulties for social workers and psychotherapists. 'Your time is up. See you tomorrow or next week' is a much less conclusive ending to a visit.

There is evidence, at least in Britain, that patients who expect a drug get one, that doctors prescribe more when they are in a hurry or when communication with the patient seems difficult, and that middle-class patients get more costly drugs than lower-class patients (Blum and Kreitman 1981: p. 170)[8]. Prescribing varies enormously between doctors and between geographical areas. Finally, the rate of prescribing varies according to how doctors are paid. In general the doctor paid by fee-for-service prescribes more than the doctor paid in other ways. This may be because patients can normally visit any doctor at any time and doctors want to make a manifest demonstration of their skill and knowledge, lest the patient try another doctor next time. Where the doctor is paid extra if an injection is given, not surprisingly, more injections are used as, for example, in Japan. In many developing countries, injections are demanded because they are thought to be more potent and quicker acting. The doctor who fails to inject is viewed as lacking in confidence. This attitude may have evolved from the 'magical' effects of the early antibiotics on many conditions which had long been prevalent, such as yaws.

The world pharmaceutical industry

Drug sales are big business and the objective is profit. The turnover of the world pharmaceutical industry was estimated at US$ 94.1 billions for 1985 (WHO 1988: p. 7)[9]. The industry is dominated by a limited number of multinational companies – most of them American. The sales of the seven leading countries are shown in Table 9.1. The 20 leading companies have 80 per cent of world drug sales (WHO 1988: p. 9)[10].

Table 9.1 **The seven leading producers of drugs by sales in 1985**

	Sales in US Dollar billions
USA	26.4
Japan	14.0
German	6.0
China	4.7
France	4.5
Italy	3.7
United Kingdom	23.

The leading exporting countries are not the same as the largest producers. They are the United States, Germany and the United Kingdom. Many American companies have branches in the United Kingdom, partly as this is seen as a convenient way of entering the markets of the Commonwealth and partly because good research staff can be purchased more cheaply.

The key to the domination of the industry is competition, not by price but by product. Initially a company's new products are protected by patent. This lasts for 20 years in the European Community, but can be extended by up to a further five years to compensate for the time taken to obtain marketing approval. During this period the product can only be sold by that company or another company which pays to be authorised to do so. Crucially, the product gets known by doctors by the snappy brand name given to it by the company, not by its cumbrous scientific name. A brand name is industrial property and a rival company using that name for its product would be stealing the original company's property. This is the key to maintaining considerable market share in the longer run. But in the United States the pharmacist is allowed to substitute a generic product for a branded product which is out of patent and there the generic market was 25 per cent of the whole market in 1992. As a result, companies making the original product have been entering the generic market with their own generics sold under a different name. Generic substitution is not generally allowed in Europe, except, with some safeguards, in Denmark.

Producing new products

The aims of each company are to produce new products which can initially shelter from competition under patent, to secure their rapid acceptance and widespread use throughout the world, to protect their invention later on by brand name, and generally to increase their share of the world market and thus their profits. The custom of the industry is not to price new drugs on the basis of cost but on the basis of what the market will bear. A new drug's price is, therefore, determined by considering the prices of existing drugs for the condition to be treated by the new drug and then adding to that price whatever the product improvement is thought to be able to command. Prices vary markedly between countries for the same product produced by the same company. Cases have been found where the price was eleven times higher in one country than another (Lall 1981: p. 192)[11]. Often it is the developing countries which have to pay the highest prices. For example, a parliamentary enquiry in Brazil found several instances of overpricing ranging from 500 to 1,000 per cent (Kanji 1992: p. 4)[12]. Over the years the industry has made exceptionally high profits (Lall 1981: p. 69)[13]. These profits arise from the fact that each product starts life as a monopoly and then becomes a near monopoly after the end of the patent period. The industry argues that its high level of profit is justified by the high risks. But a task force in the United States was 'unable to find evidence to suggest the concept of the drug industry as a particularly risky enterprise' (Task force on prescrptive drugs 1969: p. 14)[14].

The system does produce valuable new products and developing them is expensive. It is estimated that it costs about £150 million in Britain to produce a new product and get it on to the market (*Scrip* 1992: p. 6)[15]. This is because thousands of new products may have to be tried out but most of them fail to make the market either because they are found to be too toxic to be safe, or because they are found not to be as effective as hoped. Tests are carried out on animals before there are tests on humans. Research may consist of isolating natural products, applying biological theory, screening of carefully selected chemical substances, genetic engineering or simply developing a product similar to that of a rival but sufficiently different to obtain a patent. The target is the world market. Thus producing a product to treat a disease which is only found in developing countries is to enter a less profitable market than that for a disease found the world over. The developing countries, with three-quarters of the world's population, consume only a quarter of world drug production (Kanji 1992: p. 4)[16]. Companies on average spend around 10 per cent of their revenue on research and development. Part of it has to go on producing sufficient evidence to satisfy national regulating authorities that the product is effective and sufficiently safe for use as indicated to give it a licence to enter the market. The industry complains that this process can use up to 12 years of the product's patent life (Centre of Medical Research 1993)[17]. Only about 50 new chemical entities enter the world market each year out of all the research of all the companies.

Sales promotion

In the European Community, the industry spends 12–15 per cent of its turnover on promoting those products which are only able to be prescribed by doctors (Commission of the EC 1990)[18]. This is to secure rapid acceptance and widespread use. But there are obvious temptations for sales staff, within limits, to play down side effects and contra-indications and to imply wider uses for the product than are justified. A variety of methods of sales promotion are used. One is advertisements, on which most medical journals are dependent (Silverman and Lydecker 1981: p. 98)[19]. The exceptionally large number of journals marketed for doctors is due to the willingness of the industry to buy advertising space in them. No other profession is so generously served. The second method is mailed advertisements and free newspapers: it was calculated in 1976 that the average general practitioner in Britain received 50 mailed advertisements and 35 free newspapers or journals a month (Blum and Kreitman 1981: p. 160)[20]. Unless restricted, the industry is willing to give free samples (enough to treat several private patients), free gifts to doctors (deep freezes were once given away) and pay for attendance at 'conferences' held in expensive tourist resorts throughout the world, such as Davos or Bermuda. A campaign for one product cost £13.5 million and included a three-day cruise for rheumatologists on the Rhone (*Marketletter* 1991: p. 12)[21]. But the largest expenditure (two-thirds in the European Community) goes on sales representatives who visit doctors in their offices or hospitals to promote their company's products. While in Norway there is about one sales representative to 32 doctors and between 14 and 18 in Finland, the United Kingdom and the United States, there is one sales representative to every 3 or 4 doctors in Brazil and Mexico (Woodcock 1981: p. 31)[22]. In Latin America the average representative earns more than the average doctor (Silverman and Lydecker: p. 86)[23].

Sales promotion for prescribed drugs is aimed at the doctors who do the prescribing. Doctors act as agents for their patients, who cannot be expected to judge what drug is appropriate for their treatment. Patients place their trust in doctors, who are expected to judge solely on scientific criteria what drugs to prescribe. But in practice doctors are strongly influenced, not by the scientific literature, but by the skills of the different companies in sales promotion. Medical associations do not appear to be unduly concerned about this possible distortion of professional judgement.

The developed countries have in different ways tried to restrict the sales practices of the industry. For example from 1962, the Food and Drug Administration in the United States secured the right to vet advertisements for their scientific accuracy before publication, but it was never given the resources to do this thoroughly. From 1976, the Health Ministry in Britain required all advertisements to be certified by a doctor and, except in the case of repeat advertisements, to include all the details given in the statement approved by the regulating authority, and for this statement to be placed before the doctor by the sales representative. Samples were limited to those needed for recognition. Hospitality was required not to be more than doctors would buy for themselves. The amount of sales promotion expenditure which would be allowed in regulating prices and profits was restricted to 10 per cent of turnover (later reduced to 9 per cent). The industry was given the task of policing infringements of its code of marketing practices.

By 1990, most of the countries in the European Community required information sent out by the industry to be in accordance with the approved summary of product characteristics, and the majority had imposed restrictions on free samples. Some countries required advertisements to be approved in advance and in others they were controlled after issue by courts and tribunals. Still others, such as the United Kingdom, relied on the industry to monitor its own code (Commission of the EC 1990)[24]. It is reported that there were 370 breaches of the UK code in a six year period (*Scrip* 1992)[25].

In 1992, the Council of Ministers approved a directive which included requirements that:

- advertising should neither exaggerate the properties of the product nor be misleading, and should contain specified information which had to be accurate, up to date and verifiable and the selling price or indicative price had to be included (except in reminder advertisements);
- only inexpensive gifts relevant to medicine could be given to doctors and doctors should not solicit or accept any inducement;
- hospitality at meetings should be reasonable;
- samples should only be given on written request and be the smallest presentation on the market;

- sales representative should be adequately trained and should give the approved summaries of the characteristics of products when promoting them (*Council Directive* 1992)[26].

In the past the industry has been shown to have used irresponsible business methods in the developing countries – dumping time-expired or inferior drugs, selling products long banned in developed countries, using advertisements so misleading that they would have been banned in countries which regulate pharmaceutical advertising, failing to disclose contra-indications (Silverman *et al.* 1982)[27], giving financial sweeteners to doctors and pharmacists and bribes to procurement agencies. Doctors are even more in the hands of the advertisers in countries where there is very limited access to the leading medical journals. Under pressure from consumer interests and the World Health Organisation, the International Federation of Pharmaceutical Manufacturers produced in 1981 a code of marketing practices and from 1983 requested the member states of the World Health Organisation to report any infringements. What is not clear is what sanctions the Federation can apply when infringements are reported. A survey published in 1986 found that, while a number of companies had markedly improved their promotional practices in the Third World, it still found glaring differences between what companies told doctors in the United States and within the Third World. It was found that 60 per cent of undesirable promotion practices were from domestic companies and 40 per cent from multi-national companies (Silverman *et al.* 1986)[28].

The essential drugs policy and the developing countries

From the middle 1970s, the World Health Organisation became concerned about the irrational use of drugs and the inability of many developing countries to afford the drugs they needed. In 1977 the first list of essential drugs was published. In the following year, member states were urged to establish such lists. The industry stated its serious reservations about these 'misguided policies' which would 'discourage investment'. The multi-national companies had established subsidiaries in most of the larger developing countries. They held 30 per cent of the market in Egypt, 50 per cent in Argentina, 70 per cent in India, 78 per cent in Brazil and 90 per cent in Ecuador. These and other markets were at risk.

From 1979, WHO, lobbied by the consumers' movement, went further and called for an 'action programme' on essential drugs, which was established from 1981, and in the same year WHO and UNICEF agreed to collaborate on developing a system of low-cost procurement of drugs. This system, called UNIPAC, is based on Copenhagen, and supplies drugs to over 50 countries. In 1984 the World Health Assembly, the ruling body of WHO, called for activities to promote the rational use of drugs and examine the industry's marketing practices. WHO assisted countries in promoting rational prescribing, with courses and manuals for prescribers. By 1985, 80 countries had adopted the essential drugs concept.

The role of WHO did not proceed without opposition. An important issue, pressed on WHO by the consumers' movement, was the marketing practices of multi-national companies in the field of infant milk formularies. Consumers, particularly in developing countries, were being led to believe that these products were better and safer than breast-feeding, and were gradually replacing the latter. The dangers were that often the product was mixed with dirty water or the incorrect dosage was used, while milk from the breast is naturally sterilised. The result was to add to the infant mortality rate. In 1981, WHO produced the International Code of Marketing Breast Milk Substitutes. This 'interference with the operation of the free market' was opposed by the Reagan administration in the United States.

The pharmaceutical industry was also concerned that WHO was interfering with its free market and again was backed by the government of the world's largest producer – the United States. It argued that WHO 'should not be involved in efforts to regulate or control the commercial practices of private industry, even when the products may relate to concerns about health' (Silverman *et al.* 1986: p. 59)[29]. One of the issues not clarified was whether WHO intended its policies only for the developing countries or for all countries, and whether they were to apply to the private sector as well as the public sector. The consumers' movement wanted to see the policies applied in both sectors and all countries, while the industry was from 1983 prepared to accept the policy if it applied only to the public sector of developing countries. Concern about this issue was believed to be one of the reasons why the United States withheld its contribution to WHO in 1986 – about a quarter of the organisation's regular income (Kanji 1992: p. 60)[30]. Though WHO's statements became rather ambiguous, the policy was pressed only for the public sector of developing countries.

The difficulty of applying the policy only to the public sector is that the industry with its representatives' regular access to doctors, most of whom work both in the private sector and the public sector, can promote the superior quality and effectiveness of branded products, which can have three effects. First, patients using the private sector are faced with very expensive drugs which are not bought by any international tendering system but by the pharmacists from each manufacturer. The prices are seldom regulated by government. Second, the confidence of the doctors in the drugs they have to prescribe in the public sector is undermined, even if they do not actively oppose the policy. Third, the public is led to believe that the only 'good drugs' are those obtainable though private doctors. This impression is fostered by the industry's expensive packaging of their branded products. Only a few developing countries have had the courage to enforce the policy on both the private and public sector and even then products are often obtained from other countries by post.

Policy in the developed countries

As might be expected, the policies adopted by the developed countries depend to a considerable extent on whether or not the country has an industry which plays a major role in producing new drugs and selling them throughout the world. All try to satisfy themselves on the safety of products which are marketed. Norway, which is barely an exporter, limits the number of products which can be sold in Norway to 1,000. Drugs cannot be authorised for sale unless there is 'a genuine medical need' and any new drug has to be shown to be more effective than any already on the market (Lumbroso 1981: p. 75, Kanji 1992 p. 57)[31]. This compares with 36,000 brand names in Switzerland, and 15,000 in the United Kingdom and Germany (Kanji 1992: p. 3)[32]. The more drugs there are on the market, the more difficult it is to promote rational prescribing. Sweden not only regulates prices but has nationalised the distribution system. Several southern European countries (Italy, Portugal and Spain) regulate prices very tightly, based on what is calculated to be cost, and vie among themselves to achieve the lowest prices – a prize which, however, is always held by Portugal where prices for each product are fixed at the lowest among five named European Community countries (Abel-Smith 1992: pp. 125–26)[33]. France, although it is a considerable producer, regulates prices quite tightly, though it is reconsidering this policy on the grounds that it is unfavourable to the export prospects of its industry. Countries which try to regulate on cost are faced with major bureaucratic problems. No sooner has the price for one product been fixed than the industry comes out with a very similar product which will then have to have its price fixed as well.

The rationale for regulating prices is partly that new products are allowed patents and are therefore monopolised by the original producer. But more important is the peculiarity of the market situation under compulsory health insurance or a national health service. The doctor chooses, the patient consumes (or is intended to do so) and the government or the insurer pays the bill or most of it. So the doctor who does the selection of the product not only has no concern about the price but probably does not even know it. There is a complete divorce between the authoriser, the consumer and the paymaster. Recommendations have been made by official committees both in the United States and the United Kingdom to increase competition by allowing other companies to use the brand name of the original producer after the patent has expired, but in neither case have they been accepted (Abel-Smith 1976: p. 93)[34].

At the other extreme there is no price regulation in Germany or the United States, which are the two largest exporters. The United Kingdom has a different system of regulation which is based on profits earned from the National Health Service rather than on price, though companies have to apply if they want to increase their prices. The advantage from the point of view of the company is that it can shift its profits between products. Normally it will take the largest profit on its newer products which it is promoting in world markets, knowing that many countries insist that the price in their country cannot be higher than the price in the country of origin.

The role of exports also affects whether countries restrict the range of products which can be prescribed under compulsory health insurance or the health service. It would hardly help the exports of a product if it could not be obtained under the health system of the country of origin. Thus there is only a negative list of products which cannot be prescribed and paid for (largely products also obtainable without prescription) in the United Kingdom and Ireland. There is no restriction in Germany, while Denmark, Belgium and Italy (all very small exporters) have limited lists. Countries such as France and Belgium vary what the patient has to pay according to the medical importance of the product.

The governments of countries which are major world producers are faced with conflicting objectives in the policies they develop with regard to the industry. Drugs become not just a matter of health policy or of the containment of health care costs but a question of jobs and exports. If the health of the population and health care costs were the only considerations, the number of drugs on the market would be strictly limited on medical advice, as in Norway, prices would be tightly regulated and sales promotion would be banned and the drugs would be taxed to pay for an extensive postgraduate programme to keep doctors up to date on new products, their uses and contra-indications. This would be very damaging to research, jobs and exports. If the objective were to maximise the benefit to the budget, a further consideration would have to be taken into account. Exporting companies pay profits tax. If major exporters were allowed to charge high prices at home, they would be able to command high prices abroad and the tax on their profits abroad could give the ministry of finance a substantial profit even after financing the high prices for the same products when used in its health services at home. Thus these companies would be allowed high prices while those which exported little or nothing would have their prices tightly regulated. If the only consideration were exports, the level of price allowed would depend on the proportion of the product exported. If the only consideration were jobs, there would be no regulation of prices or sales promotion. There might also be a requirement that only products made in the country could be sold in the country, as in France.

Faced with these conflicting objectives, countries reach a compromise – more to the benefit of the industry in Germany than in the United Kingdom. It is because health is by no means the only consideration that policy is the way it is. And it is because of these conflicting objectives, that large developed countries do not set a good example for other smaller countries – both developed and developing – or necessarily back WHO to the hilt in placing health considerations above all others.

Policy in the developing countries

Often the prices charged by multi-national companies are greater in developing countries than in developed. This may be concealed by limiting the profits of the subsidiary company producing them in the country concerned. Transactions between the units of multi-national companies are not arm's-length transactions. What a parent company will charge its subsidiary in another country for raw materials, technical and managerial services and manufacturing know-how will depend on the policies of the different countries. These overhead costs can be used to transfer profit to another country where profits tax is low or non-existent. Thus developing countries, which have few patents of their own and therefore benefit little from the international patent system, are made to pay more than their share of the rewards to innovators abroad.

Such countries would be wise to confine their purchases to essential drugs and buy them through international tender or, if they are small, to buy them through UNIPAC or some similar agency. This would greatly reduce the number of brands on the market: in the 1970s, Brazil had 24,000 and Argentina 17,000 (Kanji 1992: p. 3)[35]. They would also be wise to require all advertising to doctors to be in line with that used in the country of origin or in a country with an effective system of control. While the concept of essential drugs is increasingly accepted, there has been much less progress in encouraging their rational use. This is because of the number of drugs on the market, the lack of continuing education in pharmacology, pressures of sales promotion and opposition by doctors to any attempts to limit their freedom to prescribe.

International action?

In an ideal world, as drug firms are multi-national, so control would need to be international, operated by the World Health Organisation on behalf of member states. Medical journals have an international circulation. It is of limited value for some countries to try to exercise tight control on drug advertising when journals from other countries in the same language are not similarly controlled. The task of ascertaining the full facts about drugs has proved a formidable task for the richest countries in the world and is beyond the resources of poor developing countries. Moreover, it is absurd for different countries to devote considerable resources to the same task. The smaller and poorer countries particularly need protection from the unethical marketing of dangerous or ineffective drugs, just as the world needs to police the trade in addictive drugs. The regulation of the world pharmaceutical industry ought to be a task given to WHO. But in view of the commercial interests of those countries which contribute most to its budget this is very unlikely to happen. Here, as elsewhere, 'he who pays the piper calls the tune'.

Notes

1   Quoted in Skrabanek, P. and McCormick, J. (1989), *Follies and Fallacies in Medicine*, Tarragon, Glasgow, p. 21.
2   Herxheimer, A. and Stimson, D.V. (1981), 'The use of medicines for illness', in Blum R. and Herxheimer A. (eds.), *Pharmaceuticals and Health Policy*, Croom Helm, London.
3   Herxheimer and Stimson (1981), 'The use of medicines'.
4   Blum, R. and Kreitman, K. (1981), 'Factors affecting individual use of medicines', in Blum and Herxheimer, *Pharmaceuticals and Health Policy*.
5   Herxheimer and Stimson (1981), 'The use of medicines', Blum and Kreitman (1981) 'Factors affecting individual use'.
6   Herxheimer and Stimson (1981), 'The use of medicines'.
7   Blum and Kreitman (1981), 'Factors affecting individual use'.
8   Blum and Kreitman (1981), 'Factors affecting individual use'.
9   World Health Organisation (1988), *The World Drug Situation*, WHO, Geneva.
10   WHO (1988), *The World Drug Situation*.
11   Lall, S. (1981), 'Economic considerations', in Blum and Herxheimer, *Pharmaceuticals and Health Policy*.
12   Kanji, N. (1992), *Drugs Policy in Developing Countries*, Zed, London.
13   Lall (1981), 'Economic considerations'.
14   Task force on prescriptive drugs (1969), *Final Report*, U.S. Department of Health, Education and Welfare, Washington D.C.
15   *Scrip* (1992), no. 1755.
16   Kanji (1992), *Drugs Policy*.
17   Centre of Medical Research (1993), *News*, January.
18   Commission of the European Communities (1990), *Proposal for a Council Directive on Advertising of Medicinal Products for Human Use*, COM (90) 212, 6 June, Brussels.
19   Silverman, M. and Lydecker, M. (1981), in Blum and Herxheimer, 'The promotion of prescription drugs and other puzzles', *Pharmaceuticals and Health Policy*.
20   Blum and Kreitman (1981), 'Factors affecting individual use'.
21   *Marketletter* (1991), 1 & 7 January.
22   Woodcock, J. (1981), 'Medicines – the interested parties', in Blum and Herxheimer, *Pharmaceuticals and Health Policy*.

23   Silverman and Lydecker (1981), 'The promotion of prescription drugs and other puzzles'.
24   Commission of the European Communities (1990), *Proposal for a Council Directive*.
25   *Scrip* (1992), no. 1755.
26   Council of Ministers, *Council Directive* 92/28/EEC of 31 March 1992.
27   Silverman, M. *et al.* (1982), *Prescriptions for Death: the Drugging of the Third World*, University of California Press, Berkeley.
28   Silverman, M. *et al.* (1986), 'Drug promotion: the Third World revisited', *International Journal of Health Services*, vol. 16, no. 4.
29   Silverman *et al.* (1986), 'Drug promotion'.
30   Kanji (1992), *Drugs Policy*.
31   Lumbroso, A. (1981), 'The introduction of new drugs', in Blum and Herxheimer, *Pharmaceuticals and Health Policy,* and Kanji (1992), *Drugs Policy*.
32   Kanji (1992), *Drugs Policy*.
33   Abel-Smith, B. (1992), *Cost Containment and New Priorities in Health Care*, Avebury, Aldershot.
34   Abel-Smith, B. (1976), *Value for Money in Health Services*, Heinemann, London.
35   Kanji (1992), *Drugs Policy*.

CHAPTER 10

Planning hospitals

Hospitals are the most costly part of health services. In developing countries, they currently account for 40 to 80 per cent of government health expenditure (Barnum and Kutzin 1992, World Bank 1992: p. 135)[1] and the higher level hospitals at the central and regional level account for 60 to 80 per cent of hospital expenditure (Mills 1990: pp. 203–18)[2]. In developed countries the range is somewhat lower. Nevertheless, the provision of hospitals needs to be planned according to the number of patients who cannot satisfactorily and economically be treated elsewhere, and the lengths of stays need to be reduced to the minimum necessary to give effective treatment. This means that, to be efficient, a hospital system needs to be planned to provide units of the right size in the right places. In developing countries it may have to be accepted that everything that could be done for patients may not be affordable. This means finding ways of establishing and enforcing priorities in the use of limited hospital beds.

An unplanned hospital system

In most countries, the majority of hospitals are non-profit organisations owned by trustees or by government, central or local. In some countries profit-making hospitals are not allowed. This may be partly out of a vague belief that making profits out of sickness is wrong or a fear that the search for profits will tempt hospitals to lower their standards. On the other hand in France, Japan and some other countries, doctor-owned hospitals or *cliniques* exist on a considerable scale. They tend to be small if they are only used for the patients of the doctor-owners whose personal reputations are intimately bound up with their hospitals. It is only from the 1970s that large commercial corporations began to develop or buy up chains of hospitals in the United States and operate them like chains of hotels. They have extended their operations to the United Kingdom

A system of private non-profit hospitals also tends to result in the bulk of them being small, even when the population is sufficient to justify one or more large hospital. This is true in Germany and other European countries as well as the United States. This may be because the funds originally raised were only sufficient to build a small hospital, or because the hospital system is reflecting the religious or class divisions of the population or rivalries between different groups of doctors. A further reason may be because the original donors wished to make provision for a particular group (e.g. Jews or women), an unmet need or a new treatment.

Hospitals which are built according to the initiatives of community groups, religious groups or the caprices of individual doctors are unlikely to result in a rational plan. Many countries in Africa and Asia have small mission hospitals sited according to the work of the religious group sponsoring it. In Latin America many cities have separate hospitals for different occupational groups owned by the social security institution serving that occupation. While many small communities may end up with too few hospital facilities, others may end up with an excess of beds. In a non-profit system, mergers seldom occur, unless strong pressure is exerted from outside. Thus in the United States, old and new hospitals, large and small hospitals, non-profit and profit hospitals struggle on side by side even though there may be an excess of hospital beds for the area – even for any stand-by need or 'option-demand'. They survive because of the affiliation of doctors with particular hospitals and the fact that, until recently, it has been nobody's business to try to secure the most favourable terms for patients. In developing countries whole wards or whole hospitals may stand empty, not because they are not needed but simply because of the lack of funds to staff and supply them.

An excess of hospital beds involves waste whether the extra beds are used or not. If used, unnecessary costs are incurred. If unused, hospitals are running below capacity and wasting some of their plant. As rates charged tend to be fixed on the basis of average occupancy, the extra costs of low occupancy are charged out to those patients who do use them, or fall on government if it is the owner.

Non-profit hospitals, like profit hospitals, are engaged in the competition for patients, unless they are already over-loaded with demand. They are also in competition for gifts and endowments. The prestige of a hospital determines the extent to which doctors want to work in it and this leads to pressure on all hospitals to acquire the latest equipment whether they have the capacity to make full use of it or not. Thus hospitals may acquire whole units which are seldom used, such as intensive care units, cardiac surgery units and transplant units, even when their staff has little experience in using them. Instead of patients being concentrated in a limited number of units planned so that each will work near to capacity and use its plant fully, patients become scattered among competing units. As a result, most specialists are denied the quantity of experience from which they could acquire high skill. The same applies to the nursing staff. A similar problem arises when social security funds have their own separate hospitals. The result is a waste of the community's resources, pockets of poor quality care and the lack of development of alternatives to hospital care. Decisions on admission and discharge are taken by doctors, and patients normally follow their doctor's advice. But doctors have not in the past seen it as their responsibility to consider the costs which they are generating for society (Abel-Smith 1976: pp. 101–5)[3].

Hospital costs

The main reason why hospitals are expensive is not so much their original construction costs, though these can seem large at the time, but their annual running costs. In the United Kingdom, these tend to amount to a quarter or a third of the construction cost: in France, a third to a half (Jolly and Gerbaud 1992: p. 3)[4].

The most common mistake that has been made in developing countries in the past is to authorise the construction of a large hospital to be paid for by some donor, or by some long-term loan without first calculating whether it will be possible to find the cost of maintaining it once it is built without distorting planned health priorities – particularly for primary care. The gift of a hospital can be a Trojan horse undermining a health plan.

The most common mistake made by some developed countries with a well-developed health insurance scheme has been to allow the unlimited construction of hospitals, whether by local authorities, non-government organisations or the for-profit sector. The hospitals are typically allowed to recover the construction cost by an annual amortisation charge included in the recurrent cost and paid for by compulsory health insurance once it is built. It is a mistake because, within limits, the supply of hospital beds determines the demand. This is often called 'Roemer's law' as it was Professor Milton Roemer who first drew attention to this phenomenon in an article published in 1959, comparing bed use in different countries and different states of the United States (Shain and Roemer 1959: pp. 71–73)[5]. Extra supply simply leads to more admissions and longer stays. A very wide range of health problems can be treated in hospitals, if beds are available. The diagnostic tests that could be undertaken on an outpatient basis, can equally readily be undertaken on an inpatient basis. There is most likely to be this unnecessary use of hospital beds if hospital care is 'free' or nearly so (i.e. paid by health insurance) to the patient while at least part of the cost would have to be paid by the patient if cared for outside hospital.

By around 1970, virtually every country in Western Europe had in operation some system of limiting centrally the number of new hospitals and extensions in each area (Abel-Smith 1984: pp. 30–31)[6]. Several countries with a substantial role played by private hospitals (e.g. France and Belgium) also authorise all purchases of major medical equipment (Abel-Smith 1984: pp. 30–31)[7]. More recently several countries (e.g. Belgium, Germany, France and the Netherlands) have devised means to put a ceiling on hospital costs by, for example, limiting the amount of income each hospital can receive from health insurance (Abel-Smith 1992: p. 129)[8].

Although hospital care is very expensive, paradoxically the purpose of a hospital is to provide a quality of care which it is actually cheaper to provide in hospital than at home. The key is quality. If, for quality care, patients need to have the services of a range of skilled personnel and access to specialised equipment, it is more economical to take the patient to where the skills are assembled and the equipment is available. If a patient needs skilled nursing, this could be provided at home, but the nurse would only be looking after one patient and three to four nurses would be needed to look after that patient on a 24-hour basis. When the patient is in hospital, the skilled nurse can look after several patients at the same time. Similarly it would be wasteful to take bulky diagnostic equipment round to patients' homes. It would in theory be possible to have a mobile operating theatre and a mobile recovery room – each loaded on a large pantechnicon which could be parked outside the patient's door. But again the equipment and the skilled staff would only be looking after the needs of one patient, while a theatre staff can process a number of patients at the same time in preparation for surgery and recovery afterwards. It is far cheaper to have patients queue to use the machine rather than have the equipment and its staff waste time in travelling and waiting for patients to be helped out of their homes to use it. Probably the last time an operating theatre was taken to a patient was when George VI had his cancer operation in 1951 in the squash court at Buckingham Palace which was hastily adapted for the purpose.

In many cases, the patient could use the skilled staff and specialised equipment of the hospital on an outpatient basis but is nevertheless admitted. There is a considerable scope for day surgery which is being significantly developed in Denmark, the Netherlands and the United Kingdom but much less in the other countries of the European Community. In some health insurance systems, such as Germany, there is no provision in the fee schedule for doctors who work out of hospital to do it, and no provision for it to be done in hospital buildings. Day surgery is more cost-effective and it has been estimated that, in the United Kingdom, one third of surgical admissions could be treated as day cases (RCS 1992)[9]. There is also potential for its application in developing countries. One private hospital in Dar-es-Salaam has diverted about a tenth of its beds for 'same day surgery'. In Colombia day surgery for hernia has been proved to be cost-effective (Shepard *et al.* 1993: pp. 136–42)[10]. In some countries 'hospital hotels' are being developed for patients who need to go daily for treatment but live too far away to go home conveniently each day. In developing countries day treatment can be provided for leprosy and tuberculosis.

The reason for unnecessary admission may simply be that space is available. Or where the same doctors look after the patient, whether it is in hospital or outside, it may simply be for the doctors' convenience, or because they would feel justified in charging inpatients more than outpatients. Particularly in the United States, a major reason for admission may be the fear of being taken to court on a malpractice charge. If anything went wrong, the doctor could argue that he or she was taking no risks and that the patient was under skilled observation.

A hospital is in part a hostel or hotel, but it is wasteful to use it as such. This is because trained staff in practice end up by doing what untrained staff could do. Unless the case is an emergency, the aim should be not to admit until most of the diagnostic tests have been done on an outpatient basis. And, once the patient is admitted, the aim is to ensure that the treatment starts as soon as possible, and that there are no bottlenecks such as waiting for the results of diagnostic tests or another doctor's opinion. If the decision-taker is solely the doctor in charge of the case and that doctor only visits on certain days in the week or is only available at certain hours in the day, there are likely to be unnecessarily long lengths of stay. Finally, discharge should be as soon as treatment is completed, provided that the necessary follow-up care is available from primary care, community services and/or family support.

Throughout the developed countries, hospital stays have been falling for many years. One reason is the somewhat late recognition that early ambulation was good for many patients after surgery. Another is the development of more drugs that are effective in combating the disease. A third is the pressure on hospitals to admit more patients. Whether this pressure is effective or not partly depends on how hospitals are financed. Does the hospital gain or lose financially by admitting more patients for shorter stays? This is discussed in chapter 14.

In the case of developing countries, one of the obstacles to reducing lengths of stay is the problem of patients admitted to hospitals with malnutrition. They could readily be looked after in a less costly institution but generally such institutions are not available. In developed countries one of the main problems in further reducing lengths of stay is the borderline between hospital provision for the aged and disabled and hostels or homes which are staffed for continuing care, not normally involving nursing care. Usually the supply of beds in the former is plentiful, while supply of the latter never appears to be adequate. The patient usually has an interest in remaining in hospital because the full costs are covered by health insurance, while the patient would have to contribute to the cost of care in a non-hospital institution. Where the hospital is paid a daily rate by insurance, it is beneficial to the finances of the hospital to retain such patients, as the daily payment exceeds the cost of care of patients who need little nursing and no medical procedures. It is, for example, calculated that 17 per cent of the patients in German hospitals could be treated in institutions outside them (Shepard *et al.* 1993: p. 22)[11].

One solution, applied in Denmark, where local authorities are responsible for providing homes for the aged, is for the hospital to charge the local authority the full costs of hospital care for patients who could be in local authority institutions, if enough places were available. This benefits the hospital because in Denmark hospitals are financed on a budget basis. And the local authority is driven to develop more homes for the aged simply because their running costs are lower than paying for care in hospital (Shepard *et al.* 1993: p. 14)[12].

Care in the patient's own home or in a special sheltered home is another alternative. The ex-patient can be given care by regular visits from nurses and, if necessary, someone can be paid to clean the home and provide meals. But if the ex-patient needs constant care, day and night, this can be more expensive to provide in the home than in an institution designed for the purpose, where staff can provide care to several people at the same time.

Economies of scale?

If, therefore, a hospital is seen as a place where skilled staff and specialised equipment are brought together so that they can be shared between patients and thus be used most economically, this would suggest that the larger the hospital, the lower the cost. The more sharing there is, the lower the cost as only some patients will need the use of particular skills and particular specialised equipment. The more patients there are, the greater the odds that all the skills and equipment will be fully used. Indeed the law of averages makes this likely. Emergency admissions become more predictable in a larger unit (Luckman *et al.* 1969)[13]. Moreover, just as a large factory makes it possible for tasks to be broken down, so that the most skilled workers only have to do the most skilled jobs, so tasks could be broken down within a large hospital with a reduction in the costs of treatment.

How far is this theory substantiated by empirical observation? Over the years many studies have been undertaken, particularly in the United States, to see whether the larger the hospital, the lower the cost. The results are confusing, as different definitions have been used for the unit of output. What is the output of a hospital? Is it services provided, cases treated, successful treatments or improvements in the community's health (Feldstein 1967: p. 145)[14]? 'Depending on the methodologies and definitions used, economies of scale exist, may exist, may not exist, or do not exist, but in any case, according to theory, they ought to exist' (Berki 1972: p. 115)[15]. Quality is important but very difficult to measure. Even if one looks at cases treated, hospitals are by no means necessarily comparable as they are likely to have different mixes of patients by disease, age and sex (McGuire *et. al.* 1988: pp. 220–21)[16]. Then, there is the further problem that it is too simple to assume that hospitals try to minimise costs so that they can compete by price in the United States. They may try and compete by perceived quality for which sophisticated equipment, irrespective of price, is used as an indicator. A National Health Service with tight budget restrictions is likely to operate under very different incentives.

In developing countries, larger hospitals have a much greater cost per day than smaller hospitals. 'Inpatient care can be up to twice as expensive in general hospitals as that in district hospitals, and in central hospitals between two and five times as expensive as in district hospitals' (Mills 1990: pp. 203–18)[17]. It is unlikely that this great difference is entirely due to a different mix of patients and the extra costs due to teaching. The larger hospital has normally been given more and better qualified staff and more equipment.

Acute hospitals are not small in the United Kingdom because it is believed that larger hospitals produce greater quality of care and economical use can be made of expensive skills and equipment. But it does appear that there are limits to the economies of scale of hospitals. These limits may be caused by a variety of reasons. Hospitals seem to become difficult to manage beyond a certain size and internal communication problems become a constraint. Moreover the larger the hospital the more difficult staff recruitment is likely to be: some staff, particularly married women, are reluctant to work far from home.

But this is to look at the problem entirely from the point of view of the costs falling on the hospital. It takes no account of the travel costs falling on staff, patients and their visitors. Nor does it take into account the difficulties visitors may encounter in dealing with a vast institution and finding out how to get to the patient they are seeking. Nor does it consider the congestion costs and car parking problems of a building housing a vast staff and receiving massive supplies and throngs of visitors.

In developing countries with dispersed populations and difficulties of travel, small district hospitals will be needed and often travel difficulties are such that a few beds have to be attached to health centres to care for less serious cases or to 'hold' patients until they can be taken to a larger hospital with greater facilities.

The classification of hospitals

Hospitals are generally classified into primary, secondary and tertiary. The exact definition of these terms differs in the usage of different countries, but in general a primary hospital is one staffed by doctors without specialist qualifications, while a secondary hospital usually has only the four most common specialties (general medicine, general surgery, paediatrics and obstetrics). A tertiary hospital has the remaining less common specialties. The greater the extent of specialisation, the greater the need for particular equipment and the greater the delegation of tasks, the greater the catchment area needed from which the more esoteric specialists will need to draw their patients, provided travel is easy to arrange.

In some countries specialised hospitals have been developed for particular categories of patients. While there are arguments in favour of isolating cases of infectious disease, it is argued that specialists in one field of medicine should not be isolated from specialists in other fields, as medical progress is fostered by cross-fertilisation of ideas. Specialised hospitals may be uneconomic if certain supporting services are only occasionally required, such as X-rays, pathology and physio-therapy, which are more economically provided on a larger scale. This may be the case with psychiatric hospitals.

In developing countries, the primary hospital may not only provide curative services on referral but provide the continuing training, guidance and supervision of the health centres and smaller units. They may also be expected to provide guidance on sanitary matters and disseminate information on disease control methods that are suitable locally (WHO 1978: p. 35)[18]. It is not easy to give responsibilities for the prevention of disease and promotion of health to institutions whose chief function is the care of the sick. This is why the orientation of the training of doctors is so important.

Normally a patient will go in the first instance to a primary hospital. Only if that hospital lacks the skills and equipment to treat the patient will referral be made to a secondary hospital and the same applies in theory to referral from a secondary hospital to a tertiary hospital. The system is advantageous for the patient and relatives, as a primary hospital can be small and therefore within reasonable travelling distance for patients and relatives. The system is also economical because it should lead to expensive skills and equipment being used only on patients who need it. If a patient who could have been treated in a primary hospital is admitted to a tertiary hospital, more expensive diagnostic tests are likely to be used to confirm the diagnosis of a common condition, simply because the facilities are available.

In practice, and particularly in developing countries, this system seldom works as intended. As high a proportion as 90 per cent of the patients treated in a tertiary hospital could have been treated in a primary hospital. This is partly because the patient knows that the tertiary hospital has better facilities and has doctors with specialised skills. The patient thus goes direct to its outpatient department in the hope of the 'best' treatment, bypassing primary care, the primary hospital and the secondary hospital. It may also be because it is known locally that the tertiary hospital hardly ever runs out of supplies, particularly of drugs, while this is much less likely to be the case at lower levels of the health care system. The third reason is that the transport to make referral systems work as intended is often not available. This means that, where there is no hospital transport, patients who are not fit to travel by bus and lack the means to hire a taxi (if either of these are available locally) has no way to take up a referral to a higher level of the hospital hierarchy. Thus the tertiary hospital becomes used by local patients with common conditions. And the costs of treating these common conditions are much higher at the tertiary hospital than they would have been at a health centre or primary hospital. For example it has been found in China that outpatient costs are 1.3 to 2 times greater in tertiary and provincial hospitals than in district hospitals (Newbrander *et al.* 1992: p. 20)[19]. When the overuse of the tertiary hospitals becomes a common practice, the primary care units surrounding a tertiary hospital are often allowed to fall into a bad state of repair and to become under-supplied, simply because they are so little used. This leads to the perpetuation of the practice of patients going direct to the tertiary hospital.

While it is politically difficult to reverse patterns of patient behaviour, there are remedies to this problem (Palmer 1991: pp. 38–40)[20]. The first is to ensure that the local primary care units and hospitals are in a good state of repair, are fully supplied, provide a friendly service and minimise waiting time. The second is to provide a similar primary care unit beside the tertiary hospital, to which all patients who are not serious emergencies or who carry referrals letters are directed. The third is to charge patients who insist on going direct to the outpatient department of the tertiary hospital, without being an emergency or a referral, the full cost of the services they use. This 'bypass charge' at least ensures that the hospital's extra costs, caused by the abuse of the referral system, are fully covered.

Planning size and location

In developed countries with good fast roads and trains, hospitals can be larger than in developing countries. In the latter, where the population is widely dispersed and travel difficult, many smaller district hospitals will be needed. As pointed out above, they are cheaper per day than larger hospitals. A compromise has to be found between being near their patients and yet not so small that they are either inefficient or ill-equipped. Small district hospitals are also needed in cities, for the care of common conditions suited for a cheaper district hospital: they can also be used for teaching. In practice, many developing countries have only the large and expensive hospitals thought essential for medical education. Once again the tail is wagging the dog at considerable extra expense. One possibility is to divide the hospital into a part performing district functions and a part more specialised, with each staffed and equipped accordingly. Or where there are enough potential private paying patients, a considerable part of the hospital can be devoted to this money-raising purpose.

Hospital design

The costs of running a hospital depend in part on how it is constructed. It may be necessary in a large city to have a multi-storey hospital because of the difficulties and the cost of acquiring a large site which would enable the hospital to be spread horizontally rather than vertically. But all tall buildings lead to substantial time used by staff in moving from floor to floor. There never seem to be enough lifts and they always seem to be in the wrong place or under repair. Where land can be acquired at reasonable cost, and this will tend to be the case in smaller urban areas, it is much better to have a hospital of three storeys which can manage without lifts or only one or two. This is particularly the case in developing countries where effective lift maintenance is much more difficult to arrange. The great advantage of ramps is that they do not need constant maintenance and repair. The costs of unskilled labour are high in developed countries and low in developing countries. It follows that hospitals should be labour-intensive in developing countries and labour-saving in developed countries.

Hospitals do not need to be built in concrete, nor is air conditioning necessary if the hospital can be designed to benefit from maximum natural ventilation in a hot climate. Nor do cupboards need to be laminated, sterilisers chromium plated or laboratories pre-fabricated. A satisfactory and safe hospital can generally be made out of local materials. The reason why hospitals in developed countries use factory-made materials, which are then assembled on site, is because making them locally by individual artisans would be much more expensive. The reverse is true in developing countries when comparisons are made with factory-made imports. Using local labour creates jobs, saves foreign exchange and can produce more personalised results – more familiar to the patients who will use the hospital.

The misuse of data on hospital costs

If rational decisions are to be made on whether it is cheaper for a patient to be cared for inside or outside hospital, when the alternatives are acceptable in terms of the quality of care available, the alternative costs of these options need to be known. This information is seldom collected or made available to clinicians taking the relevant decisions. Often the only information readily available is the average cost per treatment day. This information can be seriously misleading for the following reasons.

First, costs can vary widely per day of care. The early days are generally the most costly days as it is at this stage that diagnostic tests are done, treatment is intensive, and often the patient is dependent on nursing help with daily functions. The later days are cheaper days, because treatment is less intensive and at some stage the patient can get up, wash, make the bed and even help with other patients.

Second, costs vary greatly by type of case (Cullis and West 1979: p. 148)[21]. Patients requiring surgery may have a very expensive day when the surgery is performed because of the number of skilled staff involved and the use of sterilisers, disposables and equipment. And the cost of different types of operation also vary widely. Medical patients are likely to cost less depending on the cost of the drugs prescribed. Similarly the amount of nursing time and the number of diagnostic tests needed varies according to the treatment.

Two conclusions follow. First, to assume that discharging a day earlier will save the hospital its average cost per patient day can be very misleading. The actual saving per day is likely to be considerably below average cost in the later days in hospital, and it is this which needs to be compared with the cost of any option for caring for the patient outside hospital. Second, the incentives created for the hospital vary greatly according to different payment systems. As pointed out in chapter 14, paying a hospital per day of care creates an incentive for hospitals to keep patients for unnecessarily long stays.

Conclusion

Care in hospital is expensive and therefore its use needs to be minimised. The number of beds needed depends on the extent of admission and the length of stay. There has long been a trend to use fewer hospital beds in developed countries and many of them could go much further in this direction. This depends on making the maximum use of day surgery and providing adequate cheaper alternatives, either in other types of institution or in programmes to care for patients in their own homes. The separate financing of the alternatives represents a barrier to further progress. At least one country, the Netherlands, as explained in chapter 15, is planning to remove this barrier.

Notes

1   Barnum, H. and Kutzin, J. (1992), *Public Hospitals in Developing Countries*, World Bank, Johns Hopkins, Baltimore. See also World Bank (1993), *World Development Report 1993: Issues in Health*, World Bank, Washington D.C.
2   Mills, A. (1990), 'The economics of hospitals in developing countries', *Health Policy and Planning*, vol. 5, no. 2.
3   Abel-Smith, B. (1976), *Value for Money in Health Services*, Heinemann, London.

4   Jolly, D. and Gerbaud, I. (1992), *The Hospital of Tomorrow*, SHS paper no. 5, World Health Organisation, Geneva.
5   Shain, M. and Roemer, M. (1959), 'Hospital costs relate to the supply of beds', *Modern Hospital*, vol. 92, no. 4.
6   Abel-Smith, B. (1984), *Cost Containment in Health Care*, Bedford Square Press, London.
7   Abel-Smith (1984), *Cost Containment in Health Care*.
8   Abel-Smith, B. (1992), *Cost Containment and New Priorities in Health Care*, Avebury, Aldershot.
9   Royal College of Surgeons of England (1992), *Commission on the Provision of Surgical Services: Guidelines for Day Case Surgery*, Royal College of Surgeons, London.
10 Shepard, D.S. *et al.* (1993), 'Cost effectiveness of ambulatory surgery in Cali, Colombia', *Health Planning and Financing*, vol. 8, no. 2.
11 Shepard *et al.* (1993), 'Cost effectiveness'.
12 Shepard *et al.* (1993), 'Cost effectiveness'.
13 Luckman, J. *et al.* (1969), *Management Policies for Large Ward Units*, Institute for Operational Research Health Report, No. 1, London.
14 Feldstein, M.S. (1967), *Economic Analysis of Health Service Efficiency*, North Holland, Amsterdam.
15 Berki, S.E. (1972), *Hospital Economics*, Lexington.
16 McGuire, A. *et al.* (1988), *The Economics of Health Care*, Routledge and Kegan Paul, London.
17 Mills, A. (1990), 'The economics of hospitals in developing countries'.
18 World Health Organisation (1978), *Primary Health Care*, WHO, Geneva.
19 Newbrander, W. *et al.* (1992), *Hospital Economics and Financing in Developing Countries*, WHO, Geneva.
20 Palmer, P.E.S. (1991), 'Feeling unwell? Must you go straight to hospital?', *World Health Forum*, vol. 12.
21 Cullis, J.G. and West, P.A. (1979), *The Economics of Health*, Martin Robertson, Oxford.

PART THREE

Health services financing

CHAPTER 11

Public health expenditure and the economic crisis

During the 1980s, the cost, and therefore the financing, of health care moved high on the agenda of the discussions of health policy. The subject was discussed at the Executive Board of the World Health Organisation in 1986, at the World Health Assembly and the Commonwealth Health Ministers Conference in 1986 and was made the subject of the technical discussions at the World Health Assembly in 1987. The concern applies to both developed and developing countries. The former are concerned to find ways to contain the cost, while developing countries are concerned to maintain expenditure and, if possible, increase it to implement 'Health for All' policies.

Basic concepts

Health services can be financed either through private expenditure or public expenditure. The differences are subtle but become very important when developing countries are searching for ways to maintain or increase health service spending, while the International Monetary Fund and/or the World Bank are watching closely to make sure, as a condition of their help, that the public sector pays its way without borrowing, which could be inflationary. Put at its simplest, where services are paid for by taxes or compulsory health insurance contributions, either by employers or insured persons or both, this counts as public expenditure. Voluntary payments by individuals or employers are private expenditure. The ownership of the facilities used, whether by government, social insurance agencies, non-profit organisations, private companies or individuals is not relevant in this connection. Any of these facilities can be financed by either public expenditure or private expenditure.

This distinction between ownership (public or private) and source of finance (private or public) often causes confusion. As is illustrated in Figure 11.1, money can flow from any of the sources of finance on the left of the figure to any providers (whoever owns them) on the right of the figure.

In many developing countries, information on this important division of health expenditure has not been systematically collected. As a result, figures quoted for what countries are spending on health

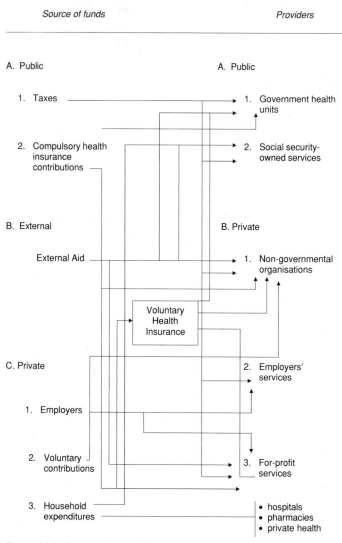

| Source of funds | Providers |

Figure 11.1 **Common flows of finance**

are often neither accurate nor comparable with those of other countries.

It is helpful to make a distinction within the health sector between expenditure on health services and expenditure on health-related activity such as water, sanitation and nutrition. One reason for making the distinction is that it is much more difficult, if not impossible, to assemble data on private expenditure on all health-related activity. Households, farms and businesses often put in their own water supply from deep wells and provide toilets for the use of the household or the staff of the business. It is not possible to isolate this expenditure from the cost of building factories or houses or developing farms. Secondly, it is not possible to distinguish what is solely expenditure on nutrition, not just because some people eat more than they need but because the foods they choose may not be by any means the cheapest way of obtaining nutrition. When calculating public expenditure, usually general food subsidies are not counted but only those aimed at the poorer section of the population and special nutrition programmes for vulnerable groups, such as young children and pregnant women. One of the most formidable problems is to draw a line, which is consistent between countries, between health institutions, caring for the elderly, mentally ill and mentally handicapped (e.g. hospitals and nursing homes) and welfare institutions looking after the same groups. The name of an institution does not necessarily have the same meaning in different countries, and some institutions perform both functions. There are many other problems in defining health expenditure. These are discussed in a manual published by WHO (Mach and Abel-Smith 1983: ch. 3)[1].

There are further problems in putting together the information on public expenditure on the health sector. One is the number of different government departments which may be spending on the health sector. If the public health sector was simply defined as what the ministry of health spends its money on, as in practice it often is, there would be major lack of comparability between the data of different countries. In table 11.1 are listed some of the government departments which may be spending money on the health sector. This list is by no means all-inclusive. There are further problems in assembling the information. The first is adding together expenditure by different levels of government without double-counting, in view of the subsidies which may be coming to local government from central government or to social security agencies or non-governmental organisations. Second, what should be included is what was actually spent during the year, not what was in the budget or what was allocated, which can be very different.

Variations in health expenditure

The study of such data as are available indicates a number of clear trends in health expenditure when figures for a number of countries are examined. First, it has long been shown that the amount which countries spend on health varies according to their level of income. The richer a country, the more is likely to be spent (Abel-Smith 1967, World Bank 1993: fig 5.1)[2]. While this is the general trend, there are several countries which spend more or less than might be expected for their level of income. Second, there is a clear tendency for public

Table 11.1 **Health sector expenditures in different government departments**

HEALTH	– may include some welfare expenditure which should be excluded;
EDUCATION	– teaching hospitals and school health;
WORKS	– maintaining the buildings used by the government health services;
DEFENCE	– armed forces' health services;
LABOUR	– occupational health services, financing medical care for those industrially injured, compulsory health insurance;
TRANSPORT	– maintaining ministry of health vehicles;
INTERIOR	– prison health services, police health services and general subsidies to local government, some of which may be used to support health services;
SOCIAL WELFARE	– health services provided to the handicapped and aged;
AGRICULTURE	– veterinary health services which protect human health;
FOOD	– nutrition services;
POWER	– free electricity for health service buildings.

Table 11.2 **Health expenditure as a proportion of gross domestic product**

Country	1971	1981	1986	1988	1989	1990	1991
Australia	5.9	7.5	8.0	7.7	7.8	8.2	8.6
Austria	5.4	8.2	8.3	8.4	8.4	8.3	8.4
Belgium	4.2	7.2	7.6	7.7	7.6	7.6	7.9
Canada	7.4	7.5	8.8	8.8	9.0	9.5	10.0
Denmark	6.4	6.8	6.0	6.5	6.5	6.3	6.5
Finland	5.9	6.6	7.4	7.2	7.2	7.8	8.9
France	6.0	7.9	8.5	8.6	8.7	8.8	9.1
Germany	6.3	8.7	8.6	8.8	8.3	8.3	8.5
Greece	4.0	4.5	5.4	5.0	5.4	5.4	5.2
Iceland	5.4	6.6	7.8	8.6	8.6	8.3	8.4
Ireland	6.6	8.8	8.1	7.3	6.9	7.0	7.3
Italy	5.5	6.7	6.9	7.6	7.6	8.1	8.3
Luxembourg	4.6	7.1	6.7	7.2	6.9	7.2	7.2
Netherlands	6.4	8.2	8.1	8.2	8.1	8.2	8.3
Norway	5.4	6.6	7.1	7.7	7.4	7.4	7.6
New Zealand	n/a	6.9	6.7	7.1	7.1	7.2	7.6
Portugal	n/a	6.4	6.6	7.1	7.2	6.7	6.8
Spain	4.1	5.8	5.6	6.0	6.3	6.6	6.7
Sweden	7.5	9.5	8.5	8.6	8.6	8.6	8.6
Switzerland	5.6	7.3	7.6	7.8	7.7	7.8	7.9
Turkey	n/a	4.4	3.5	3.8	3.9	4.0	4.0
USA	7.5	9.6	10.8	11.3	11.6	12.4	13.4
UK	4.6	6.1	6.1	6.1	6.1	6.2	6.6

Source: OECD/CREDES databank.

expenditure to grow faster than private expenditure as income increases. In other words public expenditure tends to replace private expenditure to some extent (Abel-Smith 1967, World Bank 1993)[3].

None of the data available about health expenditure in developing countries is completely comparable. In the case of the developed countries, the OECD has made a concerted effort to produce comparable data, though there has been some questioning of how far it has really succeeded. Table 11.2 shows health expenditure as a proportion of gross domestic product.

The table shows the tendency for richer countries to spend more of their resources on health, with some notable exceptions. It also shows that, after a rapid increase in the proportion of gross national product devoted to health services between 1971 and 1981, there has been a substantial slowing down in the rate of growth and in some cases the proportion of resources used on health has fallen. This is the result of deliberate policies of cost containment described in the last section of this chapter. The one country which has most notably failed to control costs is the United States. Relatively less successful have been Canada and France.

Little useful trend data over a long period is available for developing countries. But after considerable growth in health spending after the Second World War, spending has tended to fall in the 1980s because of the 'economic crisis' except in the few, mainly 'Pacific rim' countries experiencing rapid economic growth

The pressures underlying the increase in health expenditure

In the 1950s and 1960s, many developing countries were restricted in what they could spend on health services by a limited supply of trained personnel. They had not enough doctors, dentists, nurses and pharmacists to expand their services. Since then, training programmes have produced a vast increase in personnel which has removed this restriction in most of the countries. They are now limited by finance. Parallel with this increase in supply came an increase in facilities to provide the services, notably hospitals, some of which were financed from donations and loans from abroad. The developed countries were also expanding the number of doctors and rebuilding, if not extending, their hospitals. It was found that the new hospitals cost much more to run than those they replaced, partly because of the removal of bottlenecks and partly because new technology was incorporated.

A second factor has been the increase in demand in developing countries as more people have sought help from western services rather than, or in addition to, traditional services. And some increase in demand has been promoted by the services themselves as they have encouraged children to be brought for immunisation, pregnant mothers for antenatal care and ultimately for delivery, and as family planning services have become acceptable to governments and have been established as part of the health services. Demand also increased in most developed countries as the coverage of free or nearly free services expanded with the extension of compulsory health insurance. Where doctors were paid on a fee-for-service basis, extra demand was induced by the expanding number of doctors: patients were given more tests and invited to make repeat visits.

A third factor has been demographic. In the case of developing countries, the main demographic factor has been the growth of the population, mainly due to greater survival of young children. But some of the developing countries with higher income have begun to experience the factor which dominates demographic change in the developing countries – the growth in the proportion of aged people in the population. It is important because older people are much larger users of services. In developed countries, those over 65 use on average over four times more services than those aged 15 to 64 – varying from two to seven times more in different countries. Those 75 or over use six to ten times more.

A fourth factor playing some part in developed countries is the labour intensiveness of the provision of health services. While much of economic growth involves the replacement of labour by machinery, only to a limited extent does this occur in health services.

A fifth factor which applies to both developing and developed countries is the development of new technologies. More and more treatments have been developed which can be effective. The scope of surgery has widened and extended into transplant surgery. While the price of old drugs tends to fall, the price of new drugs is often very high indeed. And a vast range of equipment has been developed to assist the task of diagnosis and treatment by new techniques. These may not replace older equipment, which is still needed, but is an extra to supplement what was there already. This new equipment needs further staff to operate it. In the United States, it has been found that patients are not being given more diagnostic tests but much more expensive tests. While by no means all developing countries can afford to have all the new equipment that is available, they are under strong pressure from specialists, particularly those trained abroad, to acquire at least some of it. Parallel pressure may come from more affluent patients saying that they are willing to pay for its use. A frequent argument is that patients are having to use scarce foreign exchange to go abroad to obtain treatment which could readily be provided at home at lower cost. The difficulty with this, at first, seductive argument is that, once acquired, the government finds it very difficult, if not impossible, to restrict the use of the new equipment to those who can afford to pay. Often the difficulties and cost of maintaining and repairing the equipment, once it is acquired, are grossly under-estimated.

Finally, there is the growing expenditure on AIDS. The yearly cost of treating a person with AIDS is estimated to range from US$32,000 in the USA to US$393 in sub-Saharan Africa. While sub-Saharan Africa has 60 per cent of the HIV-infected people in the world, only 1.5 to 2 per cent of the money spent on care of AIDS is spent in Africa (*AIDS Analysis*: p. 1)[4]. The AIDS epidemic imposes formidable problems on Africa (Cabral 1993: 157–60)[5].

The economic crisis and the developing countries

The Health for All initiative could not have come at a less fortunate time. Within two years of the WHO's strategy and indicators being agreed in 1981, the world was plunged into an economic crisis. Rates of world economic growth declined. In the case of Latin America, Africa and many countries in Asia, there was actually a fall, and in some cases a substantial fall, in living standards. Between 1981 and 1983 average living standards fell by 9.5 per cent in Latin America and 11 per cent in Africa, south of the Sahara (Abel-Smith 1986: p. 203)[6]. The only part of the world where there was real growth in living standards during this period was in the East and South-East Asia, though not in the least developed countries.

The crisis also had two impacts on developed countries. First, they became acutely concerned about the rising cost of health care and searched for means of restraining them. Second, they felt unable to increase the aid they gave to developing countries. Some actually reduced it. In the case of many developing countries the effects were much more drastic. Instead of having more to spend on health care, as was hoped under the Health for All strategy, they found themselves with less. How could services be maintained, let alone expanded to meet the new agreed priorities?

The initial cause of the crisis was the sharp increase in oil prices in 1982, initiated by OPEC, the cartel of oil-producing countries. The developing countries which were not oil producers were immediately faced with a balance of payments crisis. Their exports were not sufficient to finance the import of oil at the much higher prices, in addition to other essential needs. Many developed countries were similarly placed and deflated their economies with the aim of reducing other imports so that the necessary oil could be afforded at the higher prices. This had a further effect on the balance of payments of the developing countries as the world demand for and therefore the prices paid for their raw materials declined sharply. They therefore had to export more to earn the same amount of foreign exchange. When they were unable to do this, they were sooner or later forced to devalue their currencies and seek loans from the International Monetary Fund, which in turn laid down terms which normally required a closer balance between tax revenue and public expenditure. This could most readily be achieved by cutting the latter. And the areas of public expenditure which were most often cut were the social sectors – mainly health and education; the vast spending on defence normally remained intact.

Meanwhile the oil producers were placing their large profits in the leading banks of the developed countries, particularly those of the United States and the United Kingdom. These banks in turn searched for profitable and safe investments for the funds they were holding. The developing countries became the targets for lending on a prodigal scale. It was believed that investments guaranteed by governments were bound to be safe. Often these funds were not put to use in strengthening local economies but in postponing the politically unpopular steps of cuts in living standards and public expenditure which would be the consequences of devaluation. Moreover some funds returned to the banks as secret deposits of the politicians handling the loans. Thus the strains on the balance of payments caused by the higher oil prices were followed by even greater strains in trying to pay the service charges due on foreign debts, which amounted to as much as 30 to 60 per cent of export earnings in four Latin American countries (WHO 1986: p. 48)[7]. And when devaluation was eventually accepted, these debt service payments became still larger in terms of local currency. On top of all this, world rates of interest increased, partly because of the demand from the United States for foreign funds to finance its continually increasing internal budget deficit. The developing countries needed to earn still more foreign currency to pay their way. When they could not do so, loans were rescheduled which meant that they were allowed to borrow still more to service the debts which meant that debt servicing costs became even greater every year. By 1991, sub-Saharan Africa's debts were three times higher than in 1980 and debt servicing required 30 per cent of Africa's export earnings (UN 1993)[8]. Debt amounted to 106 per cent of the region's gross domestic product (*Africa Recovery* 1992: p. 3)[9]. The chain of events surrounding the economic crisis is shown in Figure 11.2.

Devaluation worked effectively for most of the countries of Latin America. They had manufactured goods to sell as well as raw materials and could divert land from producing local foods for the home market to crops for export. At the price of much lower living standards and probably lower nutritional standards, exports were brought into line with imports. Achieving this balance was much more difficult for sub-Saharan Africa. What was called 'structural adjust-ment', by changing rates of exchange, switches the economic incentives towards exports. Imports become more expensive and the earnings of exporters increase. But most of these countries have only primary products to sell in world markets and many markets are closed by the protectionism of the First World. When they all pour more primary products on to the market, inevitably the prices go down. After plunging to as low as ever in real terms in 1991, some fell still lower at the start of 1992 (*Africa Recovery* 1992: p. 1)[10]. While

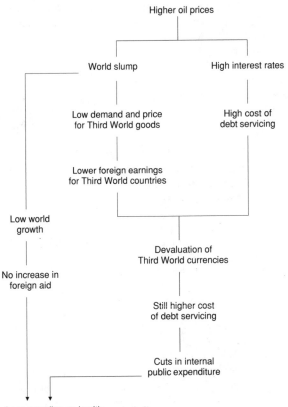

Figure 11.2 **The economic crisis**

Africa's exports have been rising in terms of quantity by 2.5 per cent a year, the prices earned for them have dropped by about two-thirds compared with 1980 so that Africa actually earned about 20 per cent less per year in hard currency in the second half of the 1980s compared with the first half (*Africa Recovery* 1991: p. 20)[11]. And in 1992, came what was possibly the worst drought in history both in the Horn of Africa, with the rapidly expanding Sahara desert, and later in western Southern Africa. Even the World Bank has admitted that a decade of structural adjustment 'has left much to be desired in terms of restoring growth and social welfare to sub-Saharan Africa' (*Africa Recovery* 1992: p. 3)[12]. The real benefits of structural adjustment were enjoyed by the developed world with cheaper coffee, cotton, cocoa, and so on.

The economic crisis had a formidable effect on the financing of the health sector. Ministers of health, committed to increase primary health care, were faced with the problem of trying to do so on sharply declining health budgets. On top of this, past programmes to increase the number of doctors and to provide the teaching hospitals for medical schools with their high running costs had matured. Other hospitals had been built with finance from foreign donors. It had seemed possible for governments to fund their running costs when the donor funds were made available, but the economic crisis made this a formidable problem on top of other demands. All these new developments were competing with the stated priority for primary health care.

Figures are not available showing how far health expenditure fell in developing countries in real terms during the 1980s. As a percentage of government expenditure, health has fallen from 6 per cent in 1985 to 5 per cent in 1990. In some countries, the share of health spending in the budget dropped by two-thirds to one half (*Africa Recovery* 1991: p. 32)[13]. But this is not a very useful way of knowing what is happening in a period when the domestic product of some countries has been falling and the budget with it, and when drugs and equipment are largely imported at much higher local cost because of devalued currencies, while on the other hand public sector wages have more than halved (*Africa Recovery* 1991: p. 15)[14]. A World Bank study of 20 African countries showed that the average publicly financed health expenditure fell from US\$9.50 per head to \$8.70 in 1985 in 1980 prices and then recovered to \$9.90 in 1987, partly due to an increase in foreign resources for the health sector. Little of value can be found from international sets of statistics (Abel-Smith 1986: pp. 202–13)[15]. The trouble is that so few countries maintain a health sector price index, which is not very difficult to do and could help ministries of health in their annual negotiations with the ministry of finance.

Ministries of health seem to respond to a decline in real resources in a similar way (Abel-Smith and Creese 1989)[16]. First the maintenance of buildings is postponed indefinitely. Second, equipment and vehicles are not repaired or replaced. Then bills are paid late. Finally drugs and petrol are undersupplied. At the same time, the pay of staff is allowed to fall in real terms. Countries appear to be very reluctant to cut staff, though those who leave may not be replaced.

At the extreme the deterioration becomes cumulative. Owing to the absence of vehicles and petrol, peripheral staff are no longer super-vised. Patient numbers fall when the supply of drugs and other essentials becomes uncertain. Staff respond to the lack of demand and the fall in their pay by spending less time at their jobs. Instead they engage in other activities to support themselves and their families, including illicit private practice. Those patients who can afford to do so use instead the licit or illicit private sector, buy drugs or herbal medicines or make more use of traditional practitioners, with the option chosen varying considerably by income group.

Despite all these difficulties there were some signs of health progress in the African region. Immunisation has reached high levels and access to safe drinking water and sanitation has improved. On the other hand, the new spectre of AIDS has developed, with 6 million adults HIV positive and full blown AIDS expected to hit one million persons in 1992 (*Africa Recovery* 1991: p. 32)[17]. This alone is a new demand of the last ten years which will require very heavy health expenditure in the future.

The reaction of an increasing number of developing countries has been to look for additional sources of finance for their health services. At first foreign aid to Africa increased from 5.8 billion dollars in 1985 to a peak of 13.2 billion in 1989 then fell to 9.5 billion in 1991 (Laishley 1992: p. 3)[18]. Indeed for all developing countries aid for health stagnated during the 1980s and as a share of total aid fell from 7 per cent in the period 1981–85 to 6 per cent in the period 1986–90 (World Bank 1993)[19]. Countries have had to look for additional resources from inside the country. One obvious source of revenue was to introduce or increase charges for public health services. Another was to develop different forms of community financing. A third was to look at the possibility of introducing compulsory health insurance. These options are discussed in the next two chapters.

The economic crisis and the developed countries

Slower rates of growth and the heavy cost of maintaining a large number of unemployed persons have led developed countries to search for ways to contain health care costs. This has become the dominant aim of regulation on top of that of asserting priorities described in chapter 6. The methods which different countries use to control costs differ according to the organization and financing of health care (Abel-Smith 1992)[20]. Where the government or the main health insurers own their health care facilities and pay health professionals on a salaried basis – what the International Labour Organization calls the direct system of financing – control is obviously easier than where health care providers are contracted by the government or the main insurers – the indirect system of financing.

Health services which are financed on a direct budget basis by government, central or local, have always been subject to cost containment, at least in theory. Overall budget financing can be applied irrespective of the share of resources collected in compulsory health insurance contributions. In theory it may seem that separate health insurers cannot be bound by this sort of restriction, but in practice they can be bound in a similar way by government using its power to restrict or veto any increases in compulsory health insurance contributions and approve any charges levied on patients, or impose reductions in or controls on the scope of the insurance offered.

Moreover budgets can be imposed on individual hospitals irrespective of their ownership even where they receive their income from different health insurers.

Cost containment can operate on consumer demand or on supply. Measures operating on consumer demand are described here as 'cost-sharing' – giving the term a wider use than is current in the United States. Cost-sharing means that the consumer has ultimately to pay part of the cost either as a user charge or as less than full reimbursement of the cost. The part falling on the patient may of course be reimbursed by supplementary insurance. This payment may be intended simply to raise revenue (and thus reduce public expenditure), to discourage user demand, or to act as a signal to the doctor or dentist authorising the use of resources that the user will have to pay and thus hopefully encourage more economical authorisation. The extreme case is where the whole cost of a particular service is borne by the user. There are further ways of trying to restrict demand on an insurance scheme. One is a no claim bonus which was, since 1989 tried out by a small-scale experiment in Germany. A second is income tax concessions to those who decide to buy services privately rather than use those they have paid for by statutory health insurance contributions or taxes. A third approach is to require prior approval for certain services, as is the case with certain auxiliary services in Luxembourg and also for certain dental procedures as in the United Kingdom. A fourth and more fundamental approach is to try to reduce the demand for health services by prevention and health promotion.

Systems of cost containment operating on supply are of a much wider variety and in recent years have taken more and more varied forms – particularly when operated on contracted services. Restriction on supply can operate on the capital stock available to insurers by limiting hospital construction or extension, closing hospitals, denial of subsidies or insurance contracts to certain hospitals, the rationing of expensive medical equipment by quota or by technology assessment. Entry of health professionals to statutory health insurance practice may be restricted or entry to medical or dental education may be limited so that there will be a reduced stock of trained personnel seeking to work for health insurance.

Current expenditure may be limited by budgets which can be reinforced by controls on the number of personnel who may be employed in the health care system. Current expenditure depends partly on the quantity supplied and partly on the price of the goods or the work-force (salaries or fees) used to supply it. Costs can be contained by operating on either. Attempts can be made to influence the authorising behaviour of doctors and dentists: they can be faced with changed incentives by altering the ratios between the payment rates for different services. Their authorising behaviour can be monitored and high authorizers warned, threatened or subjected to financial penalties. All these types of action have been taken in different countries. It is this variety of interventions which provides a long menu of options from which countries can choose.

Establishing priorities

Will measures of this kind solve the problem in the long run? Is it just putting a lid on a boiling kettle which is bound to steam the lid off in the long run? What therefore are the forces making health care costs so explosive? Much has been written about the effects of the aging population. But in the past few years the annual effect of demographic change in England has been declining and will perhaps fall to nil by 1993–4 though it will undoubtedly rise again (Maynard 1988: p. 250)[21]. In the past, the effect has been far too small to account for more than a small part of the rising costs of health care in the developed world. As pointed out earlier, the large and common feature throughout the world is the rising cost of new technology.

If health care has to be rationed what ways of doing it are there, other than by price which would be bound to be inequitable? The State of Oregon in the United States has attracted considerable interest in its attempt to establish priorities for Medicaid patients. A commission tried to work out the net added value by treating or not treating, judged by the chance of survival, the chance of cure and the chance of handicaps. The commission then corrected the list on the basis of 'reasonableness', influence of public health, the number of cases, the effectiveness of treatment and the social costs of treating or not treating (Hadom 1990)[22].

The issue has also been discussed in a report by a committee set up by the Dutch government (Ministry of Welfare 1992)[23]. They asked themselves whether the freedom and obligation of the doctor to assist the individual patient as he or she sees fit should be restricted in any way, and answered with 'an emphatic yes' (Ministry of Welfare 1992: p. 117)[24]. There should be a package of care to which everyone should be entitled, with low-priority care excluded from it. The criteria for the basic package of health care for financing by the community should be the following. First, is it necessary from the community point of view? Second, has it been demonstrated to be effective? Third, is it efficient? (Ministry of Welfare 1992: p. 133)[25]. It quotes a survey showing that two-thirds of Dutch doctors feel that 'too much manpower and resources are spent on so-called low chance medicine, that is tests and treatments, the medical result of which is slight or doubtful' (Ministry of Welfare 1992: p. 45)[26]. It calls on Dutch doctors to participate in setting up protocols, guidelines and lists for appropriate care which would be used to define by law what the Dutch health services would provide. This is a possible way forward for the long run.

Conclusion

The economic crisis has led both developed and developing countries to search for ways of increasing efficiency, finding more revenue for the health services and keeping costs under control. Many developing countries have actually had to cut their public health spending – in some cases with dire results. They have not been rescued by more health aid from the developed world, and thus have had to search for new ways of finding resources from within the country. This is the theme of the next two chapters.

Notes

1   Mach, E.P. and Abel-Smith, B. (1983), *Planning the Finances of the Health Sector: a Manual for Developing Countries*, World Health Organisation, Geneva.
2   Abel-Smith B. (1967), *An International Study of Health Expenditure*, WHO, Geneva, World Bank (1993), *World Development Report 1993: Issues in Health*, World Bank, Washington D.C.
3   Abel-Smith (1967), *An International Study*, World Bank (1993) *World Development Report*.
4   *AIDS Analysis Africa*, vol. 5, no. 4.
5   Cabral, A.J.R. (1993), 'AIDS in Africa: can the hospitals cope?' *Health Policy and Planning*, vol. 8, no. 2.
6   Abel-Smith, B. (1986), 'The world economic crisis; repercussions on health', *Health Policy and Planning*, vol. 1, no. 3.
7   World Health Organisation (1986), *Intersectoral Action for Health*, WHO Geneva.
8   United Nations (1993), *African Debt Crisis*, United Nations, New York.
9   *Africa Recovery* (1992), vol. 6, no. 4.
10   *Africa Recovery* (1992), vol. 6, no. 1.
11   *Africa Recovery* (1991), vol. 5, no. 2–3.
12   *Africa Recovery* (1992), vol. 6, no. 4.
13   *Africa Recovery* (1991), vol. 5, no. 2–3.
14   *Africa Recovery* (1991), vol. 5, no. 2–3.
15   Abel-Smith (1986), *The World Economic Crisis*.
16   Abel-Smith, B. and Creese, A. (1989), *Recurrent Costs in the Health Sector*, WHO, Geneva.
17   *Africa Recovery* (1991), vol. 5, no. 2–3.
18   Laishley, R. (1992), 'Africa faces aid cuts', *Africa Record*, vol. 6, no. 3.
19   World Bank (1993), *World Development Report*.
20   Abel-Smith, B. (1992), *Cost Containment and New Priorities in Health Care*, Avebury, Aldershot.
21   Maynard, A. (1988), 'Economic resources and ageing', in Wells N. and Freer C. (eds.), *The Ageing Population: Burden or Challenge*, Macmillan, Basingstoke.
22   Hadorn, D.C. (1990), *The Oregon Priority Setting Exercise: Quality of Life and Public Policy*, Hastings Centre Report, Hastings, no. 20, supplement 11.

23 Ministry of Welfare, Health and Cultural Affairs (1992), *Choices in Health Care*, Government of the Netherlands, Rijswijk.
24 Ministry of Welfare (1992), *Choices in Health Care.*
25 Ministry of Welfare (1992), *Choices in Health Care*
26 Ministry of Welfare (1992), *Choices in Health Care.*

CHAPTER 12

Private health expenditure

In view of the economic crisis and the real cuts in health spending in many developing countries, how to finance the health sector has become a critical issue. It is, of course, the case that many countries could use their existing resources, particularly their work-force and drugs, more effectively. But finding efficiency gains, as discussed in chapter 15, takes time and some consequential changes, such as dismissing staff, may be unacceptable.

The problem is more acute in developing countries than in developed as they cannot collect as high a proportion of their gross domestic product in taxes as developed countries. Thus public expenditure amounted to 30.1 per cent of national expenditure for a group of developed countries but only 16.3 per cent for a group of low-income developing countries (WHO 1986: p. 45)[1]. One reason for this difference is that living standards are low and taxes falling on the poorer majority would only make the poor poorer, which would be contrary to health objectives. Second, the majority of the population work in the informal sector, where it is administratively very difficult, if not impossible, to levy taxes on income. Third, taxes on exported primary products will normally fall not on foreigners but on internal producers. There may be some scope for higher taxation on imported luxuries, but the revenue is unlikely to be large. So if enough money cannot be found from taxation to support the health sector, and the government is determined to maintain the level of spending on the armed forces, where can it come from? The obvious possibilities are user charges, community-financing and compulsory health insurance. The last of these is discussed in the next chapter. But there are some less dramatic possibilities which need to be considered.

Charges which do not hit the poor

There are a number of ways of collecting extra money for the public health sector without burdening the poor with charges.

Recovery of the cost of treating industrial injury cases

The first is a charge levied on employers for the full cost of treating accidents at work. It is the normal practice to require employers to pay the cost of medical treatment for industrial injury cases, where the employer has been negligent. The employee is left to claim the compensation, including the medical costs, and if necessary go to court to obtain it. Experience from many countries has shown that an arrangement of this kind is grossly unsatisfactory. Employers or their insurance companies are in a strong position to dispute claims and very few employees can afford the cost of going to court. For this reason, the more developed countries replaced this type of provision with an industrial injury scheme which covers injury whether the employer has or has not been negligent. The employer (not the employee) has to pay contributions calculated as a proportion of earnings into a central fund. In many cases the level of contributions is varied according to the extent of risk in different occupations in the hope of encouraging employers to be safety conscious. The central fund then pays for medical treatment and rehabilitation and provides cash compensation on a continuing benefit to an injured person. If the government services were previously treating such cases, they can now obtain extra income by charging the fund.

Revenue from treating victims of motor accidents

There is an obvious logic in the cost of treating motor accident cases being made to fall on the users of motor vehicles rather than on the community in general. The simplest way of collecting the revenue is to add a sum to each vehicle licence representing the average medical cost arising from accidents from that class of vehicle. Thus the highest charge would probably fall on motor cycles, in view of the very high accident rate and incidence of serious injury. The disadvantage of this approach is that it stands out as a tax rather than as a prepayment for treatment and thus its purpose soon gets forgotten by those who pay it. Moreover even if the ministry of finance accepted that this earmarked tax should be used for the health services, it might well argue that its yield should be deducted from the annual appropriation for the ministry of health.

For this reason, and to make the new system more comprehensible to the public, it would seem better for the cost to fall on motor vehicle insurance policies. But to make this work, vehicle owners must be required to purchase comprehensive insurance policies which include provision for the cost of injuries for the driver, the passengers, persons in other vehicles involved in the accident and pedestrians. Consideration needs to be given to whether there should be maximum charges payable for the health care of injured persons. Otherwise all well-informed motor accident patients will choose the most luxurious private hospitals.

There are two possible ways of collecting the charges. The ministry of health and the insurers might negotiate an annual lump sum payment rather than incur the considerable administrative costs which would fall on both parties if each case were billed separately. The system of calculating the charges can be simplified down to an average cost per visit or per patient day. Although this system involves greater administrative costs, the money could be received by each hospital, giving it some funds which could be used flexibly according to local needs. Hospitals then have a clear incentive to submit monthly claims. It is assumed that the ministry of finance would allow public hospitals to retain the revenue. If it did not, this would remove much of the incentive for hospitals to claim.

It would be left to the insurers to decide how to recover the cost of this extra liability by higher insurance premiums. But presumably it would take these costs into account in no-claim discounts or other forms of risk-rating. In so far as this was the result, it should create some further incentive for drivers to avoid taking risks and thus contribute to road safety. The extra cost of insurance policies would depend on the frequency of accidents. In Bangkok, motor accident cases use about 40 per cent of the hospitals' resources. In Dar-es-Salaam motor accident cases were found to be only 0.5 per cent of outpatients at the large hospital to which nearly all cases were taken, so in that case, the effort may not be worth while.

Some further methods

Third, the case was made in chapter 10 for charging full cost to patients who bypass the referral system by going direct to hospitals without being referred or being a genuine emergency. This requires that the option of attending a local primary health care facility which offers free or nearly free care is readily available.

Fourth, charges for private rooms at government hospitals should cover the whole cost. In many countries they are heavily subsidised – perhaps because senior civil servants and ministers use them! Moreover they are often allowed to fall into disrepair or disuse. This may be because the medical staff resent being expected to look after patients who are paying for private rooms, away from the normal wards, but are not making any payment to the doctor. Such wards also represent competition with private hospitals where doctors can charge their patients. To obtain support for such wards it would seem right for doctors to be permitted to make agreed charges to patients. An additional advantage, from the hospital's point of view, is that the doctor is less likely to slip away to look after patients in private hospitals

Fifth, the health services can offer pay clinics out of normal working hours for those who are willing to pay and want to avoid the queues. The takings can be divided between extra payments for staff doing overtime and the health facility providing the service (see, e.g. Khallaf 1987: pp. 15–25)[2]. Some countries may of course regard such privilege as unacceptable, even though it is regularly being bought by the better off in the private sector.

Sixth, the same principle should apply in the case of dentistry. Patients should be able to make appointments for care in public facilities with part of the cost going to the dentist and the staff who do overtime.

User charges

The case for charging individual patients not using special facilities, such as private beds, has been argued on the following grounds:

- that this will prevent unnecessary or frivolous use of government services and thus ensure that the services which the government can afford to subsidise are those which are more cost-effective and that services in general are used by those in real medical need (Akin 1987: p. 26)[3];
- that as patients are paying considerable sums to private health services and to traditional services, similar charges could be made for government services;
- that in accordance with economic theory, most patients should pay at least the marginal cost of what is provided (Akin 1987: p. 26)[4];
- that charges will enable services to be improved for all users, if patients are willing to pay for these improvements (Akin 1987: p. 4)[5].

On the other hand it was been argued that charges are bound to be inequitable as no effective way can be found to exempt the poor (Gilson 1988: p. 44)[6]. Only the more developed countries can afford to operate a social assistance scheme and have the administrative capacity to do so with reasonable, if imperfect, efficiency.

Frivolous use

The argument that patients make unnecessary or frivolous use of services assumes that people can always tell whether use is necessary or not. Second, it assumes that charges will deter the unnecessary user. Both assumptions are very questionable. Many patients are in no position to know whether their symptoms are serious or not. Third, the relationship between fee increases and frivolous use was investigated in Swaziland and no evidence was found of any relative decline in frivolous users. The greatest drop in utilisation was in immunisation and preventive services which was against the government's intentions (Yoder 1989: pp. 35–42)[7]. Finally, the use of services is seldom without cost. It is often tacitly assumed that the only costs of using health care are any charges which may be levied by providers. But an important additional cost is time away from other activities which can be very important not only for those who lose cash earnings when away from work but also for subsistence farmers and, not least, mothers taken away from their household duties. A further cost is that of travel for some patients. All these costs can be very large indeed in developing countries.

Patients pay for private health services

A recent study investigated choice between government and mission hospitals in Tanzania by interviewing a population sample of over 1,800 living in range of both (Abel-Smith and Rawal 1992: pp. 329–41)[8]. The respondents stated very firmly that the problem with mission hospitals was that they were expensive. Those who could not afford them went normally to the government hospitals. The two are thought of as serving different markets.

The argument for charging full cost to those who can pay

The classical economist's argument that prices of government services should move upward to the full cost with exemption for the poor and subsidies for the near poor was stated firmly by the World Bank in its 'Agenda for Reform' (Akin 1987)[9] – launched at a press conference during the World Health Assembly. The central argument was that preventive services benefited the whole population while curative services benefited only the individuals concerned. Thus subsidy should be concentrated on the former. This, of course assumes that free preventive services will be fully used, even if curative services are subject to charges. In practice, curative services often have the indirect effect of securing cooperation with preventive services. What was never made clear was whether the World Bank was advocating the denial of services to those who were thought able to pay but said they lacked the current resources to do so. Or was the policy to be one of treating first and seeking to recover the money afterwards. In this case, it would be bound to lead to the problem of debts, which would be very expensive to collect. One admission to hospital could consume half a family's annual income, even though the family had substantial assets in the form of land and animals.

Surveys show that the decisions to seek heath care and who to consult are caused by many factors – hours of service, travel time, waiting time, the availability of doctors or of drugs and the way patients are treated, but price is also important (World Bank 1993: p. 70)[10]. Not surprisingly charges will normally reduce the demands on the health services and those whose demands are most reduced are likely to be the poorest. The extent to which this is so depends on the level of the charge (see, e.g. Bethune *et al.* 1989: pp. 76–81)[11]. High charges can lead to the waste of health resources when under-occupied staff have little to do. An initial large drop in demand, as in Ghana, may be followed by a considerable recovery (see, e.g. Waddington and Enyimayew (1989): pp. 17–47, (1990): p. 287–312)[12].

If the yield of the charges has been successfully used to improve services, the composition of the user population may have changed. The better-off may have switched back to the government health services, disguising a much larger drop in demand by the poorer section of the population. The evidence on the effect of user charges is admirably summarised in a recent paper by Andrew Creese (1990)[13]. He concludes that increasing reliance on direct payments makes 'access harder for the poorest – and neediest'.

How much revenue can be raised from charges? Creese suggests that the experience of the poorest countries in Africa suggests an average of about 5 per cent of operating costs (Creese 1990: p. 5)[14]. But this makes no allowance for the administrative cost of collecting the charges. Fee revenue from hospital charges in three Latin American countries varied from 1 per cent to 8.5 per cent of recurrent expenditure (Newbrander *et al.* 1992: p. 29)[15].

All the European Community countries have at some stage used modest cost-sharing to reduce demand but it has not been by any means the most important mechanism for cost containment (Abel-Smith 1992)[16]. Moreover, the poor are normally protected through social assistance schemes. The impact has been relatively small, except perhaps in France and more recently in Portugal, both as a revenue-raising measure and as an attempt to control demand directly or indirectly.

Exempting the poor

The fundamental difficulty with any system of charges is how to exempt the poor. To argue that those who can afford it should pay the full cost of the curative health services they use and that differential fees should be used 'to protect the poor' (Akin 1987: p. 3)[17] is fine in theory but extraordinarily difficult, if not impossible, to apply in practice in a developing country. Some mission hospitals may seem to be able to do this, but where they are most successful is where staff have served in a community for long periods and the mission has extensive contact and knowledge about local families as the result of its other work. Traditional practitioners are also able to collect charges, but they also have close links with the community, are often willing to accept payment in kind and wait until resources are available to pay them – at harvest time.

Moreover it cannot be stressed too strongly that willingness to pay is not necessarily evidence of ability to pay. People may be able to lay their hands on money in what seems a crisis rather than face the humiliation of claiming exemption. But this does not mean that they do not go without before harvest time or before the next pay comes in or later get into a spiral of debt at high rates of interest and even end up by selling some of their land. In Tanzania it was found that 60 per cent of households had borrowed, pawned or made special sales to pay health care bills (Abel-Smith and Rawal 1992)[18] (see Table 12.1). Most use of health services is by women for themselves and their children and they seldom have command over all household resources.

*Table 12.1   **Means of raising money for health care in last year for those who have used these means***

	Number	*Percentage*
Borrowing from relatives/friends	648	35.6
Selling animals	303	16.6
Selling farm produce	588	32.3
Selling valuables	274	15.1
None of the above	732	40.2

Those who claim that it is practicable, in a developing country, to 'target' charges only on those who are not poor need to be able to point to an example where such a system works with tolerable accuracy. At present it seems that a system of granting discretion to health staff is bound to result in very rough justice, if not corruption and favouritism. Whatever the rules, it seems, from several studies (e.g. Mills 1991: pp. 1241–52)[19] and the author's experience of many countries, that in practice exemption is seldom granted. Certificates of indigency from village leaders can be subject to political or kinship bias and cannot be operated effectively in urban areas. And a formal system of means-testing by workers trained for the purpose, the cost of which is only justified in the case of substantial bills for hospital care, can result in substantial bad debts from those who are assessed as able to pay in whole or part. Moreover the fact must be faced that it is formidably difficult to assess the means of those who work in the informal sector or subsistence agriculture as most people do in the poorer developing countries. And there is in many cases the further complication of determining who really constitutes the household in societies which are polygamous in law or practice.

At least three countries (Costa Rica, South Korea and Thailand) operate systems by which poor people can apply annually for a certificate or card which entitles them to free health care. None of them succeed in identifying all the poor. The card in Thailand has been systematically investigated. The cards are issued to 14–20 per cent of the population. One study showed that only 60 per cent of card holders were poor and that 17 per cent were wealthy (GTZ 1988: p. 32)[20]. Despite this failure of targeting, it is nevertheless true to say that such systems are easier to administer where relatively stable families are the norm, as is the case in all three of these countries. The possibility of applying such a system was investigated in Jamaica but not implemented. One of the problems was that of defining the household.

Such evidence as is available leads to an inescapable conclusion. Generalised systems of charging are bound to face problems of equity[21]: some of the poor are likely to be made poorer when charges are introduced in a health system which has deteriorated into a situation where supplies are insufficient for it to function properly.

Charging to improve services

What about the fourth argument for charges – that it enables services to be improved for all users? Its importance depends on how far services have deteriorated. A recent study in Tanzania found that the main complaint people had of the government services was that drug supplies ran out (Abel-Smith and Rawal 1992)[22]. Drugs supplied by Danish aid (DANIDA) arrived at the beginning of each month in rural areas; these supplies tended to run out by the fourth if not the third week of the month. Respondents were asked where they got their drugs and what they paid. A considerable proportion of drugs were not bought at the same health facility. This was particularly the case with government services where over 26 per cent were bought outside the facility – mainly at chemist's shops (see Table 12.2)

Table 12.2   **Where medicine obtained after consultation (percentage of positive answers)**

Place of purchase	Following consultation at		
	Government	*Mission*	*Private*
Same health facility	73.6	95.6	93.5
Another health facility	1.5	0.8	0.0
Chemist shop	21.0	1.3	3.2
Other	3.8	2.3	3.2
TOTAL	99.90	100.00	99.90
Number of positive answers	(808)	(385)	(186)

Finally, respondents were asked what they paid for the medicines or treatment. The replies for those who had used government health facilities are shown in Table 12.3.

The average amount paid was Tsh 671 (about 3 US dollars) with a very wide dispersion: 5 per cent paid Tsh 2,000 or more (over 9 US dollars). The number of payments reported was 248 which can be compared with the 213 respondents who had used these services but had obtained their drugs elsewhere. This suggests that 35 of the paying respondents (14 per cent) had made illicit payments for drugs at the government health services.

In these circumstances a charge for each drug of (say) Tsh 50 (20 US cents), if it could lead to drugs always being available, would

Table 12.3   **Cost of medicines prescribed at a government consultation**

Cost	Number	Percentage
Up to Tsh 49	23	9.3
Tsh 50 up to Tsh 99	17	6.9
Tsh 100 up to Tsh 199	27	10.9
Tsh 200 up to Tsh 399	49	19.6
Tsh 400 up to Tsh 999	84	33.9
Tsh 1,000 up to Tsh 1,999	35	14.1
Over Tsh 2000	13	5.2
TOTAL	248	99.9

MEAN OF PAYMENTS MADE – Tsh 671

reduce the cost of buying drugs in the private sector for people who became sick towards the end of the month even if the system of trying to exempt the poor was far from effective. When the population of Tanzania were asked in the survey what they would be willing to pay if drugs were always available, there emerged substantial support for this policy (Abel-Smith and Rawal 1992)[23].

Which items should be subject to charges?

The advantage of charging for drugs is that the patient receives the consultation before the question of payment is raised. The patient can be told how important it is to have the drug dispensed and that, for example, economising by ordering half the prescribed dose of antibiotics, as often happens in some developing countries, would be counter-productive. This last practice is avoided by making the charge flat rate rather than a proportion of the cost. It is also advantageous to charge per item on the prescription rather than per prescription form. This makes the prescriber think carefully whether further items are really needed.

There is also a rationale for charging for delivery of babies as it is an event which can be predicted. Thus money can be saved up to make the payment. An additional reason is equity: rural mothers have to pay traditional births attendants, as a western service is not available locally, while urban mothers can use local hospitals without payment. There is also a case for charging for services which can be postponed until the money is available to make the payment. This is the case with most dentistry. A low charge per day to cover the cost of food provided in hospital is often accepted without complaint but it is often a fallacy to argue that when a family member goes into hospital, the family is better off. This takes no account of the costs of travel to hospital for the patient and the relatives.

The level of charges

The level of charges depends partly on what alternative means there are for finding extra money for the health sector, and partly on how far the health services have become depleted. If they are set too high, they can be a serious deterrent to use. On the other hand, if expenditure on services is reduced to such an extent that they are spurned by many of their intended users, the aim of equity will not be achieved. It is better to make services acceptable to their potential clientele, than to force the latter into the private sector where they are likely to pay much more than for public services, even if the latter went so far as to charge full cost. Thus a balance has to be struck between concern for the poor, bearing in mind that any attempt to exempt them is likely to result in rough justice, and concern for the majority who could afford to pay considerable charges for acceptable public health services.

The World Bank is right to point out that charges are likely to be collected much more assiduously (and possibly too assiduously in the case of exempting the poor) if the money is retained locally and spent on the improvement of local services. But this is easier said than done. First, there is the problem of seeing that the money is not misappropriated. Some countries place the money under the control of committees of local people. This is a good basis for building local participation. But there is still the problem of where the money can be safely deposited if there are no local banks. Second, there is the logistic problem of finding a way for distant health units, which do not have functioning transport, to use the revenue to purchase drugs and other supplies.

The introduction of charges requires careful preparation and planning which cannot be rushed. First, the population needs to be informed about the purpose of charges. In some countries, for example Kenya and Uganda, the adverse reaction to the introduction of charges was so strong that the charges were abolished by a decision taken at the highest level soon after they were introduced. Second, the procedures for handling the money have to be carefully worked out, forms (such as receipts and daily records) have to be designed and printed and staff have to be recruited and trained. The administrative costs of operating a charging system should not be underestimated. In some small health units they can be larger than the revenue likely to be collected.

Community-financing

Introducing charges at government health services creates an incentive for communities to organise informal prepayment schemes, under which those who pay contributions become once again entitled to free health care. The advantage of all types of insurance is that it is less of a burden to pay regularly when well, than to pay suddenly when sickness strikes. The prospects of making this operate successfully are greater when payments can be made through a producers' cooperative which deducts the contribution before paying the producers for their produce. There are many isolated examples of prepayment schemes operating in different types of community. What is not clear is how long they last and how much they depend on unusual charismatic leadership.

It is hard to find an example of a country which has managed to develop prepaid community-financing into a national system. A country which made a substantial effort over seven or more years to develop such a system in the rural areas is Thailand, where user charges are considerable. Cards were sold which provided the family with six to eight free treatments for episodes of illness during the year. Volunteers were carefully selected by the villages and extensively trained. There were incentives for villages to promote the system as part of the premiums were retained in village health funds. But despite the relatively low level of premium (4–6 US dollars for a family for a year) and the high priority given to the programme by the Ministry of Health, coverage was less than a quarter of the population in the implementation areas (GTZ 1988)[24]. Moreover those who joined tended to be the better-off and those with above average health risks. It has still to be shown that voluntary local prepayment schemes can make a major contribution to health financing, except perhaps in a coercive political system. This may not, however, be their main purpose which may be to develop greater participation in health matters at the local level – a step towards empowerment.

Informal health insurance is, of course, only one of the many types of community-financing. Others are extensively discussed elsewhere (e.g. Abel-Smith and Dua 1988: pp. 95-108)[25]. One common initiative is a revolving drug fund. An initial supply of drugs is provided to the community by the government or some donor such as UNICEF. The person selected by the community to be in charge of the fund then charges the local population for drugs according to use. The revenue thus obtained is used to replace supplies, so hopefully the system can continue indefinitely. Whether it does will depend on the efficiency of the management and whether the revenue collected is sufficient to buy new supplies which may have gone up in price. Experience has shown that the managers of such funds need training, not only in the correct uses of the drugs they will be handling, but in book-keeping and pricing. Moreover, while a volunteer may be willing to do this without payment for an initial period, a share of the proceeds is likely to be needed to secure a continuous service. One advantage for the local community is that basic drugs are made available conveniently in the village at prices lower than they could be obtained in the private sector. If other health services are available outside the village, those who use the revolving fund are saved the time involved in going outside the village for their simpler health needs.

This type of initiative was sponsored for African countries by the Regional Committee of WHO meeting in Bamako in 1987 with strong support from UNICEF. Its aims included accelerating the development of primary health care with priority for women and children, encouraging community mobilization, decentralisation, making the community principal partners of health development and ensuring a regular supply of the most essential drugs (Jarrett and Ofosu-Amaah 1992: p. 166)[26]. It was hoped that primary health care would become self-sustaining. The success of the 'Bamako initiative' was evaluated in 1992. The evaluation showed a variety of payment mechanisms, variable quality improvements, differing mark-ups on the drugs sold, problems of access for the poor and only some potential for sustainability (McPake *et al.* 1992)[27]. There have been complaints of unrealistic demands for management and logistic support, the burden falling on the poor where there is a high mark-up on the drugs to cover staff costs, and the perverse incentives to encourage curative rather than preventive care (see, e.g. Kanji 1989: pp. 120–20)[28].

Profit-making private health insurance

Some have suggested that the spread of private insurance can take a noticeable load off government services. At present this plays an insignificant role in the poorer developing countries. Even where it does have coverage of around 5 per cent of the population, the cost of the premium limits further expansion. As experience has shown, particularly from the United States, private insurance has costs which do not fall on a compulsory public programme – not only profit but sales promotion costs. Another factor pushing up costs is the fact that those who choose to be insured are likely to be less healthy than those who do not. Insurers protect themselves with a whole series of limitations in the policy. A further problem is that each individual insurer is in ·a weak position to negotiate favourable prices from suppliers or to require participating doctors to observe a list of essential drugs. Thus they are generally reimbursing patients for part of their bills which may be padded with unnecessary services, where the supplier knows that most of the cost will ultimately fall on the insurer. The potential contributor is not only faced with high premiums but flat-rate rather than earnings-related premiums which is generally the practice in compulsory schemes. On top of this, those who would wish to cover their families have to pay substantially higher premiums to do so, which generally means that coverage of dependants is low. Finally, preventive services are often not covered by the insurance, as those who pay the premiums are not believed to attach importance to them.

Conclusion

Charging for health services is one way of finding more money to support the health sector. Some charges can be introduced which do not fall upon the poor. In the case of other charges, the case for introducing charges depends on the actual position facing particular public health services. If they have deteriorated to such an extent that they lack essential supplies and even the poor have to resort to the private sector to obtain them, it is more equitable to charge than not to charge, even though the attempt to exempt the poor is likely to be far from fully effective. This is assuming that the revenue can be used to make adequate supplies available. In such circumstances the poor can no longer afford 'free' health services.

Notes

1   World Health Organisation (1986), *Intersectoral Action for Health*, WHO, Geneva.
2   Khallaf, S.E. (1987), 'Economic and financial constraints and their impact on health provision in Egypt', *Financing Health development*, WHO, Geneva.
3   Akin, J. *et al.* (1987), *Financing Health Services in Developing Countries: An Agenda for Reform*, World Bank, Washington, D.C.
4   Akin *et al.* (1987), *Financing Health Services.*
5   Akin *et al.* (1987), *Financing Health Services.*
6   Gilson, L. (1988), *Government Health Care Charges: Is Equity Being Abandoned?*, EPC Publication No. 15, London.
7   Yoder, R.A. (1989), 'Are people willing and able to pay for health services?' *Social Science and Medicine*, vol. 29, no. 1.
8   Abel-Smith, B. and Rawal, P. (1992), 'Can the poor afford free services: a case study of Tanzania', *Health Policy and Planning*, vol. 7, no. 4.
9   Akin *et al.* (1987), *Financing Health Services*
10 World Bank (1993), *World Development Report 1993: Issues in Health*, World Bank, Washington D.C.
11 de Bethune, X. (1989), 'The influence of an abrupt price increase on health service utilisation: evidence from Zaire', *Health Policy and Planning*, vol. 4, no. 1.
12 Waddington, C.J. and Enyimayew, K.A. (1989), 'A price to pay: the impact of charges in Ashanti-Akim district, Ghana', *Health Planning and Management*, vol. 4, no. 1, 17–47 and Waddington and Enyimayew (1990) 'A price to pay, part 2: the impact of charges in the Volta region of Ghana', *Health Planning and Management*, vol. 5, no. 4,.
13 Creese, A.L. (1990), *User Charges for Health Care: A Review of Recent Experience*, Current Concerns No. 1, SHS, WHO, Geneva.
14 Creese (1990), *User Charges.*
15 Newbrander, W. *et al.* (1992), *Hospital Economics in Developing Countries*, WHO, Geneva.
16 Abel-Smith, B. (1992), *Cost Containment and New Priorities in Health Care*, Avebury, Aldershot.

17   Akin *et al.* (1987), *Financing Health Services.*

18   Abel-Smith and Rawal (1992), 'Can the poor afford free services?'

19   Mills, A. (1991), 'Exempting the poor: the experience of Thailand', *Social Science and Medicine*, vol. 33, no. 11.

20   Deutsche Gesellschaft für technische Zusammenarbeit (GTZ) (1988), *The Health Card Programme in Thailand*, Munich.

21   For a much fuller discussion of the question of equity, see Gilson (1988), *Government Health Care Charges.*

22   Abel-Smith and Rawal (1992), 'Can the poor afford free services?'

23   Abel-Smith and Rawal (1992), 'Can the poor afford free services?'

24   GTZ, op. cit., p. 36.

25   Abel-Smith, B. and Dua, A. (1988), 'Community-financing in developing countries: the potential for the health sector', *Health Policy and Planning*, vol. 3, no. 2.

26   Jarrett, S.W. and Ofosu-Amaah J. (1992), 'Strengthening health services for MCH in Africa: the first four years of the 'Bamako Initiative', *Health Policy and Planning*, vol. 7, no. 2.

27   McPake, B., *et al.* (1992), *Experience to Date of Implementing the Bamako Initiative: a Review and Five Country Case Studies*, London School of Hygiene and Tropical Medicine, London.

28   Kanji, N. (1989), 'Charging for drugs in Africa: UNICEFs Bamako Initiative', *Health Policy and Planning*, vol. 4, no. 2.

CHAPTER 13

Compulsory health insurance

Nearly all developed countries use compulsory health insurance contributions in whole or part to finance their health services. The Central and Eastern European countries are replacing their government-financed health services with insurance schemes, or are planning to do so. And owing to the economic crisis, more and more developing countries are contemplating, planning or initiating such schemes. As most countries in Latin America already have compulsory health insurance, though in many cases coverage is low, the recent trend is towards developments in Asia and Africa. Thailand has recently introduced a scheme and schemes are being considered in Malaysia, Indonesia, Papua New Guinea and Vietnam in Asia and Nigeria, Tanzania and Zimbabwe in Africa. As in the past in developed countries, all schemes start by covering compulsorily only those in regular employment, because of the difficulty of ascertaining the earnings of those in informal employment and because many of them cannot afford contributions with no employer to share the cost.

The advantages of compulsory health insurance

Compulsory health insurance has a number of potential advantages as a way of financing health services:

- In most countries that have compulsory health insurance schemes, the insured, with the help of their employers, can pay the whole cost of the services they use, not just a small part of the cost which in practice is all that user charges can collect. It is administratively much easier to identify those with regular jobs and make them and their employers pay than find those who are poor to exempt them from charges. Employers benefit because insured persons obtain quicker access to services and avoid the queues and delays in the public sector. They also hopefully obtain a healthier work force.
- Health insurance contributions provide a relatively stable source of income which cannot be diverted for other purposes without an explicit change in the law.
- Experience elsewhere has shown that ministries of finance have not attempted to cut the health budget, because health insurance has been introduced. And there are obvious advantages in a source of

revenue which is largely independent of the ministry of finance; this is one reason why this option is so widely supported in Central and Eastern Europe.

- Health insurance can bring in money to pay for better health services for all to use. The more people choose to use their insurance for the private sector, the shorter the queues at public health services and the fewer people there are to share the limited drugs and other supplies that can be afforded in the public health services. And if the insured want to use the public sector, they and their employers pay the full cost.

A compulsory scheme has substantial advantages compared with a voluntary scheme operated by private insurers. First, compelling people to join by law saves the cost of sales promotion. Indeed if the collection of the contributions is combined with another social security scheme, there would be virtually no additional administrative cost of collection. Administrative costs would only be involved in securing the provision of the benefits. Second, the scheme can be designed to provide preventive and curative services from the same health units. Third, a unified scheme is able to exercise bargaining power with providers and obtain services on favourable terms and negotiate arrangements for paying providers which do not give incentives for the provision of unnecessary services. These options are not available to a small employer and are often not exploited even by large employers. Finally the scheme avoids risk-rating and thus has the following social advantages:

- Risks are spread between those with high needs for health services and those with low needs. No one can be sure in advance into which group he or she may ultimately fall.
- Those in healthy occupations, such as office workers in insurance companies and banks are made to cross-subsidise those in occupations subject to greater health risks.
- The cost of covering dependants is spread among those currently with none and those with many.
- The higher paid cross-subsidise the lower paid by contributions related to earnings.

These are the four key principles of 'solidarity' or equity which should govern compulsory health insurance schemes. They explain why no country uses unregulated private insurers to provide the scheme. If employers were simply required to take out defined insurance for their employees and their dependants, the premiums paid by employers of clerical staff (such as banks or insurance companies) would be much lower than those in hazardous industries. Also, employers would be tempted to seek to hire single persons and to sack them on marriage or the birth of a child. It is, however highly desirable that dependants are brought in at the start of the scheme.

This focuses attention on longer-term costs. It is easy enough to devise a scheme which is affordable only for insured persons. Some countries have done this and then found they could never afford to bring dependants into the scheme on the same terms.

The only compulsory scheme which abandons these principles of 'solidarity' is the system developed in Chile by the Pinochet military government. All those in employment, formal or informal, have to pay 7 per cent of their earnings for health insurance. For the lowest income groups, under-financed public health services are available. The insured above the lowest levels of income are able to obtain free primary health care from the public sector but have to pay 25 per cent of the cost or, if their earnings are a bit higher, 50 per cent of the cost for hospital care. But the disadvantages of using the public sector are that standards are low, drug supplies run out and there are long waits for certain treatments. This income group also has the option of using private sector primary care by buying vouchers obtainable from the office of the statutory insurer. Providers participating in the scheme can place themselves on one of three levels of charges. According to the pricing bracket chosen by the provider, the scheme will pay, on behalf of the insured person from 30 per cent to 50 per cent of the fee. The higher the fee level, the less the scheme will pay.

Those with still higher earnings and good health are allowed to use their 7 per cent of earnings to purchase a private insurance scheme. Premiums are adjusted according to risk and those with pre-existing medical conditions will not be accepted as members. The limitations of coverage are defined in each insurer's policy. Any employees who join must cover all their dependants under the same conditions. Thus premiums vary according to family size. Those who join are generally required to pay 10 to 40 per cent of the cost of each service they use. There are tax concessions to encourage people to select this type of insurance. Employers can deduct 2 per cent of earnings from taxation for those joining a scheme and the insured person's contributions are tax deductible.

This model defies the basic principles of equity or 'solidarity' in the following ways:

- the compulsory contributions of the high paid are needed to subsidise the lower paid.
- all the insured should have access to the same services.
- all providers should be paid on the same basis for all insured.
- tax concessions for private health insurance and high co-payments are unacceptable.

It was to avoid 'family size rating' as well as 'health risk-rating' that, when compulsory health insurance was introduced in Europe, standard contributions were generally introduced for all employees and employers.

The practicability of compulsory health insurance

A health insurance scheme needs not only to be desirable in principle but practicable in the particular circumstances of the country concerned. These circumstances are listed below.

1. There must be enough persons to cover with insurance

To make it worth the effort, there must be enough persons working for employers on a regular basis (not paid daily) outside the public sector to make the scheme viable and to take a noticeable load off the public health services. While the private sector may be small, those working in it may nevertheless make extensive use of the more expensive public services because they tend to work in the main cities. Unless contributions were wholly paid by employees, covering public employees involves extra costs for government in its capacity as employer.

2. The services provided must be sufficiently attractive

It must be possible to provide insured persons with services which they regard as worth paying for. To work effectively health insurance should be designed to be self-policing to a considerable extent. Employers comply with the law and pay over both their own and their employees' contributions because employees want to enjoy the benefits of being insured and employers appreciate the advantages of healthy workers. It is vital that employers and employees should accept the services as a substitute for any existing arrangements which employers may have made for the health care of their employees – at least for the vast majority of employees.

A scheme would be unlikely to work effectively if insured persons were offered exactly the same services as were available to those not insured. The insured can be given advantages in a number of different ways including access to doctors in their own private offices or special clinics for insured persons at separate times or on separate premises. If public hospitals have several classes of ward, patients can be given access to a higher class or the option of using a contracted mission or private hospital. It may at first sight seem inequitable to give insured persons privileges, but it is possible to confine the privilege to amenity and convenience, and not to the quality of care.

3. The scheme must be affordable

The scheme has to be affordable by employers and employees – even eventually in small and vulnerable enterprises. It would be perverse to establish a scheme which had the effect of bankrupting employers and creating further unemployment. There could be adverse effects on some small firms, if large firms which already provided good health services for their employees exercised pressure and were allowed to contract out.

4. The country must have the administrative capacity to operate the scheme efficiently

The country must have the administrative capability to operate the scheme with efficiency and without corruption. An accurate and up-to-date record has to be maintained of those entitled to the benefit and they alone should use the designated services. Administrative costs need to be kept as low as possible and the cost of the benefit needs to be regularly monitored and kept under control. Providers have to be paid without delay. The success of the scheme will depend on the management capacity of those who are put in charge of it. For many countries, the introduction of health insurance has been one of the most complex administrative tasks they have yet attempted. Political support at the highest level is needed to see that the scheme is able to attract the key personnel to run it and that the considerable start-up costs are fully met. But the administrators should be appointed for their managerial competence, not their political loyalty.

5. There needs to be a firm commitment to 'Health for All'

The government needs to be fully committed to the World Health Organisation's 'Health for All' principles. There is a danger that once the more vocal section of the population (those with regular jobs) are provided with acceptable health services, there will be less political pressure to improve and extend services for those who are not covered. This has happened in some countries in the past. But if a government intends health insurance to be a step towards 'Health for All', the money released by the scheme will be redeployed to strengthen the public health services. It is important that both the insured and the non-insured should use the same services to a substantial extent. As the World Bank points out 'services designed only for the poor will almost inevitably be low-quality services and will not get the political support needed to provide them adequately' (World Bank 1993: p. 70)[1].

6. There must be enough trained personnel

There must be sufficient trained health workers in the country to provide the service without robbing the services available to the rest of the population of staff which they can ill afford to lose. If prompt access to doctors is essential to make the scheme acceptable to employers and employees, then there must be enough underemployed doctors to make this possible. Moreover the income which can be obtained from health insurance must not be so large that it leads key staff to leave the public service and makes it even more difficult to persuade staff to accept posts in the remoter rural areas. The starting point for fixing rates of pay should be earnings in the public sector. Doctors with established private practices may well argue that the amount they would be paid (whatever the system of payment) is derisory compared with potential earnings from private practice, while underemployed doctors will silently rejoice at the prospect of a reasonably reliable income. This is an area where concessions cannot be made without dangerous consequences. One possibility in a developing country is to relate the amount of insurance practice doctors are allowed to provide to their period of previous rural service.

Types of health insurance fund

There are many ways in which the scheme can be organised. One possible way of achieving the objective is by employers' liability, rather than by insurance. In other words, a legal obligation is placed on defined employers to provide or secure the provision of defined health services for their employees at the employers' cost. Such laws were a common feature of colonial development. They tended to be applied to enterprises in remoter areas such as agricultural estates of different kinds (e.g. sugar or tea estates, rubber plantations or mines). This approach is still used in some African countries. The advantage is one of simplicity. It does not require much in the way of a new administration. All that is needed is some system of seeing that there is compliance with the law and that the services are up to the required standard.

There are, however, a number of potential disadvantages in this approach:

- Employees may not trust such services. The 'doctor' may be seen as working for the employer rather than for the patient by refusing to sanction time off work and turning a blind eye to industrial diseases.
- There is bound to be substantial inequity in such arrangements. Financially secure and paternalistic employers will provide good services, while financially insecure and unsympathetic employers will provide the minimum needed to appear to satisfy the legal requirements.
- An employer with well-paid staff can provide good services at a low cost in terms of the proportion of the pay roll, while employers of low paid staff may have to pay a higher proportion of pay roll to provide services which are much less good.

A second possibility is to have one insurance fund covering all the insured, run by a parastatal whose board is appointed by the government, though powers may be delegated to local areas. This simplifies administration when people change employer or the place of residence.

A third way is for a series of local funds run by joint committees of employers and employees to bring control nearer the consumer and avoid direct government control which can lead, in some countries, to political appointments and corruption. Cross-subsidies will be needed between richer and poorer areas to create equity.

A fourth pattern found in such countries as Germany, Japan and South Korea is a system of insurance largely based on industry, which was the way in which health insurance developed in those countries. Under the law all funds have to provide certain defined benefits: some other benefits may be optional. Within the regulations, employers and employees can jointly control their own schemes. The trend, over the years, has however been to amalgamate insurance funds to prevent any of them being too small to achieve economies of scale. Decentralisation to a number of separate funds gives the advantage that unions can negotiate for extra benefits beyond those which the law requires. And joint control between workers and managers may help to secure more harmonious working relationships. But it does not necessarily lead to much competition between funds. Nor does it lead to tight control over costs. Indeed insurers have nearly always found it necessary to negotiate prices and contracts with providers through a federal organisation. It has, moreover, been found that control over price but not quantity is far from giving control over total costs.

A fifth possibility is to have competition for members between highly regulated funds with a central body collecting the contributions and distributing them among the chosen insurers according to the risks of their members, as recently proposed for the Netherlands and described in chapter 15 below.

While all these options are viable, four key principles should not be overlooked. First, the minister of health should retain power to approve the level of remuneration of health professionals to ensure that it is not allowed to become so high as to damage recruitment and retention in the remaining public health services. Second, persons who could be insured should only be compelled to pay contributions in areas where adequate services are available for insured persons to use, without damaging the public health services provided for the non-insured. Third, what must at all costs be avoided is allowing the scheme to be controlled by providers. Inevitably their interests will take precedence over those of insured persons. Fourth, government must exercise tough control on administrative costs which can escalate due to bureaucratic inefficiency.

Types of health insurance system

Health services for the compulsorily insured are not left to the functioning of the unregulated free market because two vital elements for the functioning of such a market are missing. The first is informed consumers who know precisely what they want to buy. Second, the functions of authorising purchase and supplying it are not separated. Doctors and dentists do both. For these reasons, governments intervene in a variety of ways to try to secure value for money. Health systems differ according to the bodies who do the controlling and regulating – central government, local government or the insurers who pay the bills. Often a complex mix of regulators and controllers has emerged according to the political traditions, historical experience, and power groups within each country. And it is because of these differences that a system which works well in one country cannot simply be transferred to another and produce the same good results. Each country must make its own choice, taking into account the likely behaviour of the different actors.

An insurance agency has a wide variety of options for securing the availability of services. It is not possible to make a comprehensive typology of systems of organising national health insurance as most are complex mixes of different types of provision. At one extreme are the direct systems with salaried professionals and usually their own hospitals and health centres. This model is to be found not only in several Eastern European countries (though many are currently changing it), but in Greece, Portugal and many countries of Latin America. At the other extreme are countries using the indirect method where health insurance funds contract all services paying private doctors on a fee-for-service basis. This is the pattern in Belgium, Canada, France, Japan, Luxembourg and Germany. It does not follow that the insurers are left alone to get on with the job. Central government plays a very active regulating role and is constantly intervening with new measures in the attempt to contain costs and secure value for money.

In Denmark, the Netherlands, Italy and the United Kingdom general practitioners generally work in their own offices and are paid on a capitation basis or some variant of it. The hospitals used are owned by local government in Denmark, mainly by central government in the United Kingdom and by a mix of public and private agencies in the other two countries. Sweden has local government hospitals and the option of primary care from free local government health centres with salaried doctors or private fee-for-service paid doctors where the patient has to pay part of the fee.

Another way of delineating systems of national health insurance is to show who has the power to decide what within each system. Who decides the number of insurance funds, how are the members of each fund selected, who chooses the providers, the prices and the scope of the packages of care? Some of these decisions may be taken by government (central or local), some by the funds, some by the providers or by the insured persons themselves.

Some criteria for choosing among options

The decision between the many alternatives which have developed around the world will depend on the importance attached to the following considerations.

Choice and competition

In virtually all developing countries, people who can afford to do so are already making choices between health units in the public and private sectors. They will want choice to continue under health insurance and to be widened for those who cannot currently afford to use private sector services. Competition between providers puts pressure on providers to make their services as acceptable to users as possible.

Quality

All services should, as far as possible, be up to the required standard at the start of the scheme and measures should be taken on a continuing basis to see that quality is maintained. In the past, it was often argued that this could only be achieved if the services were under the direct control of the insurer by using the direct method of provision. But there are ways of imposing quality on independent providers. Quality assurance can be judged at three levels. The outcome of the treatment is the ultimate test but it is very difficult to assess. A less rigorous test is by process. This has two parts. The first asks did the doctor do what he or she ought to have done (history, proper examination, tests where necessary, rational prescribing of treatment, tissue tests, etc)? One approach to this is by examination of the medical record. The second asks was the service convenient and acceptable to the patient? Was there difficulty in getting an appointment, what was the waiting time for the consultation and obtaining the prescription, what was the attitude of the doctor as perceived by the patient? This can be ascertained by random questionnaires or from complaints. A less rigorous test, which is easier to apply, is to lay down in advance criteria for the setting. Were the building equipment and staff adequate for the job?

Simplicity of administration

The scheme should be as easy as possible for both patients and providers to use. Administrative costs need to be kept to a minimum.

Prevention and health promotion

Health insurance can be adapted to encourage personal preventive services by financial incentives. If extra money is provided for each personal preventive service provided (e.g. immunisation, family planning or cervical screening), health professionals will find it worth their while to make special efforts to send for those who ought to come and keep a register of who has come and who has not. A stronger financial incentive is lump sum payments for achieving different levels of coverage.

Health promotion can be encouraged by a regulation requiring all health insurance funds to spend a specified proportion of their income on health promotion. Part of this can be spent on health promotion literature (including a magazine for members and information on environmental and workplace risks). Part can also be spent, for example, on counselling on nutrition, exercise or the excessive use of drugs and alcohol, courses for people wanting to stop smoking, on how to cope with stress, or on dental hygiene. Sports clubs can also be subsidised. Part can be directed to health education in schools or for elderly people. Special allocations can be made for environmental health and early rehabilitation.

Economy

Unnecessary services should not be provided, there should be incentives for economy and opportunities for fraud should be minimised both in the case of providers and users. The following are some of the ways of making services cost-effective:

- Covered persons should have access to only one chosen primary care provider at a time. This prevents the covered person shopping around among different providers for treatment for the same illness.
- Specialist and hospital services should only be covered on referral from the chosen primary care provider.
- If there are separate insurance funds, insured persons, to whichever fund they are attached to, should have access to the same hospitals. Separate hospitals for each fund, which have been developed in some countries, are bound to lead to under-utilised facilities, duplication of expensive equipment and inconvenience for patients and visitors.
- Only a list of essential drugs should be paid for under the scheme.
- Wherever possible prices should be negotiated, not just imposed by the provider.
- The use and cost of services should be continuously monitored to compare utilisation patterns and identify the more costly authorizers of services for administrative action.

- The payment system of providers should not create incentives for excessive or unnecessary services. This critical issue is discussed in the next chapter.

Introducing a scheme

Preparing a scheme may well take several years and cannot be hurried for the following reasons:

First, an administrative agency or agencies will need to be established or adapted and the composition of the controlling board or boards decided, members appointed, staff appointed, equipment selected, ordered and installed for financial control and monitoring usage. Staff will need substantial training.

Second, establishing a system of collecting contributions, if it does not exist already, is by no means easy. Where there is no income tax, it will be very difficult to create a system of collecting compulsory contributions from the self-employed.

Third, contracting providers, selecting and defining payment systems and contract terms and negotiating initial rates of payment can be a time-consuming and contentious operation.

Finally, establishing in advance the information system needed to monitor utilisation, and costs and quality is also a further major task.

Conclusion

It will be clear from the above that establishing a health insurance system can be a formidable administrative task. Moreover the transition from a direct service to a system of contracting requires careful planning. As a system adapted from experience elsewhere may not work well in a new context, there is a very strong case for trying out new models in one local area before applying them nationally. Special measures are needed to make national health insurance compatible with Health For All principles. It is not just a matter of securing insurance but of regulating the way in which, and the price at which services are provided. Establishing a central mechanism for collecting the money does not rule out consumer choice between suppliers to generate efficiency.

Notes

1 World Bank (1993), *World Development Report 1993: Issues in Health*, World Bank, Washington D.C.

PART FOUR

Controlling costs and securing user-friendly services

CHAPTER 14

Methods of paying providers

The system of paying providers has a major influence on the cost of services and also on the attitudes of providers to users.

Doctors

Doctors are required by the ethics of their profession to do the best they can for the health of each patient. Their treatment should therefore be independent of the system by which they are paid – or indeed whether they are paid or not. But in practice, doctors, like everyone else, respond to financial incentives.

In many societies it was the practice for doctors to have a 'normal' fee which they reduced for those unable to pay it. And in some cases bills would not be paid for long periods or would never be paid. The normal fee would vary according to the reputation and training of the doctor. This type of system still operates in many countries both for 'Western' and traditional doctors. Health insurance challenges this by wanting to pay the same fee to any doctor for the same service. Naturally the doctors with high reputations do not want to see their fees standardised downwards. While a scheme has a low coverage of the population, the prestige doctors can practise outside it. The challenge comes when coverage becomes large. This underlying issue has led to confrontations between insurance schemes and doctors in many countries in the past. Often governments have felt it necessary to intervene to stop services being suspended to insured persons by a doctors' strike or boycott.

Where doctors have been in a position to assert their case with legislatures, a number of solutions to this dilemma have been found. One such solution was to exclude the higher income groups from insurance as in Germany where they have to buy their own private insurance. Another was to allow certain designated doctors to charge more, as is the case in France. A third solution was to allow specialists to charge more than a general practitioner for giving the same service, as in Belgium. A fourth was to have an entirely different payment structure for specialists, as in the United Kingdom, which offered very high pay to a limited number of doctors.

This underlying tension forms the background to the discussion of different ways of paying doctors set out below.

Reimbursement

Without negotiated rates

Under this system, providers fix their own charges and the patient is reimbursed in full or for only a proportion of the charges. Thus the larger the reimbursement, the more providers may be encouraged to raise their charges and increase their services. This is the opposite of cost containment, but not unwelcome to doctors for obvious reasons.

A more common system, but usually under private health insurance, is for the insurer to reimburse at standard rates laid down in the policy. This also encourages providers to raise charges and increase services. This is what has happened over many years in the United States. For this reason very few countries use this system under compulsory health insurance. It does, however, operate for some doctors in France and under the Medicare scheme for hospital insurance in the Philippines. When the scheme began in 1972, it was reimbursing 70 to 100 per cent of hospital costs. Owing to higher prices and the inclusion of dependants, by 1982 the proportion of costs covered had fallen to 48 per cent for primary care hospitals, 30 per cent for secondary hospitals and 15–18 per cent for tertiary hospitals. Moreover, the admission rate rose from 3 per cent per year to around 6.5 per cent per year, partly because care outside hospitals was not covered (Patag 1983)[1].

With negotiated rates

Where reimbursement is used, the compulsory insurance scheme normally tries to negotiate charges with associations representing providers and expects them all to observe them. There is often a continuing conflict with those providers who refuse to observe the contract negotiated by their association. This has been the experience of France over many years. There was a similar conflict with doctors in Canada until finally a federal law in 1984 led the province to pass laws specifying that no reimbursement would be given to the patient unless the doctor charged at the negotiated level. Naturally patients would avoid any doctors who placed themselves outside the scheme in this way.

It is because of these problems that most compulsory health insurers pay direct to providers contracted rates agreed in advance by negotiation. These rates cannot be exceeded. Any charges or co-payments which can be levied on patients also form part of the contract. Such contracts can take a variety of forms.

Any system of reimbursement has the disadvantage that the patients have to find the money to pay for services before they can claim reimbursement. Poorer people may find this difficult and so hesitate to use the services. On the other hand, patients do see the bill which shows how much the insurer is paying on their behalf and this also limits the extent to which a doctor can charge the insurer for services which were never given which became a problem in Belgium in the early 1980s (Glaser 1991: p. 230)[2]. An exception is in the case of diagnostic tests where patients may not know what tests were in fact done on their blood.

Payment of the doctor by the insurer

Salary – the direct method

There are obvious advantages in the direct method. Doctors can, in theory at least, be deployed where they are needed, trained to use resources economically and to have a strong preventive orientation. But it is a system designed by saints for saints and most countries do not have enough saintly doctors to operate it as intended.

In many Latin American countries, and also in Central and Eastern Europe, doctors arrive late and leave early. Long waits for treatment are often due to trade union practices as well as bad time-keeping. Doctors insist on seeing only three or four patients an hour and may even refer up to a third of them to specialists inside the health centre which involves another long wait. The pharmacy, because of late-arriving doctors, has suddenly to start its work two or three hours late, which again leads to further waiting time for patients, after the first few patients have had their prescriptions dispensed. This makes the service not only unpopular with its users but expensive for the contributors. And where the doctors use the service to recruit the better-off patients for their licit or illicit private practice after working hours, getting satisfactory health care involves the patient in further wasted time in the evening.

Patients often complain of lack of common courtesy under this system of payment. This may be due to low morale among the doctors, as well as hurrying to get away to do the 'real job' of private practice. In many countries there is no choice of doctor: patients are told which doctor they will see. It is not very satisfying professionally for doctors to spend time with patients whom they never expect to see again. And it is not surprising that many doctors come to see themselves as working for the director of the service in which they are stationed much more than for the patient.

In addition, and this particularly applies to Eastern European countries under the old regime, it becomes the custom to make payments not only to the doctor but also to the nurse. These payments are much too large to be called tips. They have different names in different countries. They vary from 'gratitude payments' in Hungary, to 'the top left-hand drawer' or 'the brown envelope' in other countries. The money is given by patients determined to obtain the best attention and resources in what is nominally a free service. Such practices inevitably disadvantage the poorer patients. Indeed many of them find they cannot afford to use the 'free' services provided for them by the beneficent health planners, because they cannot offer this extra money. It is because of this corruption, the under-financing of the services, and the fact that the services are far from being user-friendly that all the Eastern European countries are determined to get rid of the system as soon as possible. In many cases, they argue that their services functioned much better under the old days of health insurance.

What has been the experience of Western Europe? The three continental countries which have salaried doctors in primary care – Spain, Portugal and Greece all suffer from some of these problems in varying degrees. What about the more northern countries? Doctors are not salaried in primary care in Britain, Denmark and Norway, and are no longer in Finland, so this leaves the jewel in the crown – Sweden. And now even that jewel has become a bit tarnished. It came as a great shock to the health planners of Sweden with their beautiful health centres to discover that the upper-middle income groups refused to use them and started going to local doctors in their own private offices and simply paying them in full for their services in the old-fashioned way. One difficulty with the health centres was that you seldom saw the same doctor twice. This was because a doctor, after working at night, was given two days off. From the beginning of 1992, some politicians have decided to turn the doctors in the health centres into entrepreneurs. They are now given budgets out of which they have to buy the hospital services for their patients.

A system to be avoided is part-time salaries (e.g. for four-hour sessions) for primary care doctors. Those countries which have used this system have found it subject to great abuse. Doctors are tempted to take many four-hour sessions at different health centres and rush their work at each one of them. They become under particularly strong pressure to arrive late and leave early.

A salaried service more often works successfully in hospitals. It is generally applied to all doctors from the leading specialists and professors down to the housemen or interns. Thus it is considered successful in Germany, the United Kingdom, in the public hospitals of France and other countries of Europe. There are no plans to change it. In some cases the specialists can supplement their salaries by treating patients on a paying basis in special private wards or private hospitals. The disadvantage of this is that a 'dual track' may develop, as in the United Kingdom. Many of the higher income groups do not use the national health service for specialist and minor hospital services (although they still have to pay their share of the costs). They prefer to take out private insurance so that they can have private rooms, more choice of time of admission for non-emergency care, and the knowledge that the specialist whom they have chosen will be directly responsible for all their hospital care rather than delegating some of it to junior doctors. It is notable that there is hardly any 'dual track' in Denmark or Sweden. Everyone is content to use the public hospitals.

Fee-for-service

This system is used in such countries as Canada, Australia, New Zealand, Japan, South Korea, Belgium, Western Germany and Norway. In several of these countries it was adopted because the doctors refused to participate in a scheme which paid them on any other basis. The advantage for the doctor is that it gives him or her the flexibility to increase income by providing further services. Payment is for work done. The disadvantage is the time needed to record and claim for each service and deal with queries raised by the insurer.

The advantage for the patient is that it can provide complete free choice of doctor, general practitioner or specialist, for each illness or even during the course of the same illness. In practice the system encourages patients to go direct to the specialist and this is expensive because specialists tend to order more diagnostic tests than general practitioners. If the doctor has access to a hospital, the patient can be treated by the same doctor in and out of hospital. The doctor has incentives to make the services attractive, prompt and courteous. There is, moreover, no incentive to under-provide. As a result, the insured person will find the premium high because of the high utilisation it encourages.

While the insurer derives satisfaction from contented users, the disadvantages for the insurer are escalating costs due to growing utilisation and the administrative cost of monitoring claims. Under negotiated standard fees, the only way doctors can augment their income is by providing more services, and this they are in a position to do. In Ireland, until recently, there were only two fees – one for a home visit and the other for an office call – but the doctor could still encourage repeat visits. When the fee schedule includes some 2,000 medical acts as in Germany or in South Korea, the doctor can provide more technical procedures and order more diagnostic tests. Some procedures are bound to be particularly high earning for the doctor for the time involved and this will encourage their use. For example, diagnostic tests were identified as a problem in Belgium and Germany, until the relative payments for them were reduced. And where the doctor has purchased a particular piece of medical equipment, there are strong financial incentives to use it so as to pay off the capital cost as soon as possible. This has been a special problem in Western Germany. Now costs are contained by fixing a budget for all technical services provided by all doctors under statutory health insurance. If the number of medical acts increases, the rate of payment for each goes down proportionately.

Repeat visits may lead to further prescriptions. There is evidence that doctors paid on a fee-for-service basis tend to prescribe more drugs (Abel-Smith and Grandjeat 1978: p. 26)[3]. This is one of the reasons why Italy changed over to a capitation system of payment for all general practitioners. If the doctor dispenses the drugs prescribed, as in Japan, making a profit on every drug and particularly if paid extra for injections, there are major incentives to over-prescribe and give injections, as mentioned in chapter 9 above.

A fee-for-service system is more open to fraud than other systems of payment. Services can be claimed that were never given. Sometimes this is in collusion with the patient who shares the fee. Or else doctors use the insurance numbers of patients whom they have treated before and simply make claims for further services. If proper control is not exercised, claims can be made for patients who are dead or never existed – 'ghost patients' as they are called in Latin America.

Concerns about quality can arise in a number of contexts. Where doctors are paid on a fee-for-service basis for surgery, there is the possibility of some of it being unnecessary. A much quoted study of the United States showed that varying geographical rates of surgery seemed to be explained by the number of surgeons in each geographical area (McPherson *et al.* 1978: pp. 273–88)[4]. Doctors may be tempted to undertake surgical procedures of which they do not have recent experience. Patients, who can visit several doctors during the course of an illness and receive drugs from each, may take them in a dangerous combination.

To try to limit these problems, the insurer needs to monitor claims closely and maintain statistics of each doctor's usage ('doctor profiles') to ascertain which doctors make high claims and in what respects. Sanctions may be applied against high-claiming doctors. Claims may be queried when the procedures appear inconsistent with the diagnosis, if this is disclosed, which doctors refuse to do in France. Moreover there is always the possibility of fraud either from patients (such as cashing prescriptions at the pharmacist for cosmetics) or from doctors (such as colluding to share the profits with a laboratory for pathological tests which were never done). An alternative way of limiting over-utilisation is to require prior approval for hospital admission or surgery. All this makes such systems expensive to administer. Moreover, while fee-for-service payment may at first sight appear to interfere least with the clinical freedom of the doctor, it may end up interfering far more than under any other system of payment.

A further way of keeping the cost under control is to make the patient pay part of the cost. In South Korea, outpatient visits rose from 4.8 per person per year in 1980 to 7.4 in 1985. Only when co-payment was more than doubled was the increase checked. But by that time the patient was required to pay 65 per cent of the cost of an outpatient visit (Kim 1987)[5]. This considerably reduced the value of the insurance which it was originally intended to provide. Co-payment has, however, a negligible impact on usage in France where most people take out private insurance which reimburses the co-payments.

Capitation

Under this system doctors are paid a negotiated sum per month for each person who chooses to register with them for primary care, whether that person uses the service or not. A patient can normally only visit that doctor until the insurer is notified of a change to another doctor. Thus there is very substantial continuity of care. Access to specialists is restricted to cases referred by the general practitioner, except in emergency, and this helps to keep down costs. Under most systems, the doctor has responsibility for the listed patients 24 hours a day and 7 days a week, though a deputy can be appointed by the doctor for some nights and weekends. Many do this by a rota with neighbouring colleagues. The doctor is not allowed to see a listed patient on a private payment basis.

This system has long been used in a pure or modified form in Denmark, the Netherlands, and the United Kingdom and from 1980 in Italy. It is also used in Finland and Indonesia and more recently in Ireland (replacing the simplified fee-for-service system) as well as Costa Rica. It is also used in some health maintenance organisations in the United States.

The advantage for patients, compared with using a salaried doctor in a health centre, is that they have their own personal doctor whom they have chosen (up to the limits imposed on doctors' list sizes). This doctor has continuous responsibility for the patient's care outside hospital. When the patient is sent to hospital, the general practitioner receives a report from the hospital with recommendations for the later care of the patient. The disadvantages are that patients cannot go direct to a specialist and that another doctor takes over their care if they are sent to hospital. The general practitioner may also have poorly equipped and poorly furnished premises as in a pure capitation system doctors have to pay for the upkeep of their premises out of their capitation payments.

The advantage for the doctor is having the right to run the practice in whatever way seems best. The only paper work, other than the maintenance of patients' medical records, is to report additions and departures from the list of patients. The only limitation on clinical freedom is that prescribing may be monitored by the insurer. If the doctor is a member of a partnership, this has been by choice and the partners have agreed to work together and decided what supporting staff they will employ and what they will be paid. The disadvantage for doctors is that the maximum permitted list size may be achieved by their early 30s and then, unlike other professionals, they cannot increase income except through the negotiation process which affects all doctors. Moreover a doctor who wants to combine general practice with hospital work will find it hard to do so.

The advantage for the insurer is that the cost is predictable, though the cost of the doctors' prescriptions is not, if they are separately paid for. Moreover capitation payment does create some incentive for doctors to be evenly spread in relation to the population. There is also some incentive for doctors to adopt a preventive approach where they think it will save them time in the long run. Doctors and patients are likely to be reasonably content and there is a simple answer to a dissatisfied patient, which is to try another doctor. Administrative costs are low as all that is needed is to keep records of which doctor should be paid for which patients and operate a procedure for dealing with complaints or to sanction doctors who break the crucial rule that doctors cannot see their own listed patients on a private paying basis. There may be worries about doctors with poor premises or the overuse of deputies or excessive referral to specialists. But evidence from countries where it is used shows that the latter is not in practice a major problem with the system.

A pure capitation system can be modified to take account of special problems. For example, higher capitation payments can be paid for elderly patients, allowances can be added for seniority, for working in remote areas and attendance at continuing education. The doctor's rent can be reimbursed to encourage spacious premises which can then be made subject to inspection. Fees or target bonuses can be paid on top for defined preventive work, as in the United Kingdom, or for each visit made by patients, as in Denmark.

Conclusion on doctor payment

All this leads to three conclusions. The first is that it is very difficult to make a hierarchical salaried service put the patient's convenience first. The second is that at least the higher-income groups, if not all income groups, want choice – at least in primary care. They want to be treated as customers and not as patients. If they do not like the service, they want to be able to take their custom elsewhere. And they want to know that, if they do, the doctor they leave will suffer not just in his or her pride but financially as well. The cash nexus keeps even health professionals on their toes. And this is true whether the patient does the paying or the insurer on his behalf. Finally, no system will work well if the doctors think they are seriously underpaid.

Hospitals

There are four main ways of paying the hospital, though there can be variations within them and ways of combining more than one method.

Allocating a fixed annual budget which cannot be exceeded

Budgets can be given not only to hospitals owned by the service but also to privately owned hospitals, as in Canada. While a budget gives a hospital director incentives to use it most effectively in purchasing supplies and hiring staff, what it does not do is to give any incentive to encourage doctors to reduce lengths of stay to the minimum needed for effective treatment. If there are patients waiting to come in, shorter lengths of stay will lead to more admissions. As the early days of treatment are the more costly for the hospital, the shorter the length of stay, the larger the budget required. The incentive of the manager is above all else to keep expenditure within the budget allocated. Therefore, where there are patients waiting for admission, reductions in lengths of stay or the introduction or extension of day surgery place this objective at risk (Beech and Morgan 1992: pp. 133–48)[6]. Pressure can be put on managers by closing adjacent hospitals, but this may only result in longer waiting lists. The problem can be eased by supplementing the budget by a payment for each admission as in Massachusetts, but a standard payment per admission may create perverse incentives such as to prefer medical cases to surgery cases or to admit patients simply for diagnostic purposes. To adjust according to the types of patients admitted would make the system complex to operate. An alternative is to take into account the work done last year in fixing next year's budget.

Payment by itemised bill

This system is normally used by private hospitals billing private patients. Whatever the costs are, they can be passed on to the patient with profit added. The obvious disadvantage is to encourage escalating costs on a scale even greater than payment of the doctor by fee-for-service. While the level of charges for each item can be negotiated, the doctor responsible for the patient is in a position to order more and more tests and undertake more and more procedures. The temptation to behave in this way is likely to be greatest when the doctor owns the hospital. The insurer is in a weak position to question afterwards how much was really necessary.

Payment by a daily rate

Many countries in continental Europe have for many years paid hospitals on an inclusive daily basis covering all costs, even that of the doctors. While this gives the hospital an incentive to economise, it has the serious drawback that it encourages long stays because the later days of stay are less costly for the hospital. Every hospital wants to accumulate a surplus, if possible. This would be called profit in a for-profit hospital or a way of financing developments, such as purchasing new equipment, in the case of a not-for-profit hospital.

This can be countered by the insurer employing doctors or nurses to visit patients in hospital and review the possibility of early discharge. Or the insurer can state the number of days allowed on admission according to diagnosis: the hospital has to request permission for further days from the insurer.

Payment by diagnosis

This system was developed first in the United States and adopted for use under the health insurance scheme for the aged – 'Medicare'. Diagnoses are grouped in some 470 categories, based partly on cost and partly on medical similarity, to give the system credibility with the doctors who use it. A lump sum is paid to the hospital for the whole period of stay. Several European countries have been working on systems for use in their own countries. The system has the advantage of cost control, as payment is related to output, and it removes the incentive for long stays. It clearly provides strong incentives for diagnosis before admission and early discharge. Indeed the incentive to discharge may be too strong, so that very frail patients are sent away without being sure that they will be properly looked after. There are also incentives for discharge and readmission a day or two later to claim a second payment, though a computerised system can be designed to pick up such cases and refuse payment unless there is clear justification for this having happened. A third risk is what has become known as 'diagnostic creep'. Where there is more than one possible diagnosis, the doctor is expected or trained to choose the one which brings a higher payment to the hospital. Indeed the whole system depends on the honesty of the doctors who state the diagnosis. In some countries, such honesty could not always be relied upon, particularly when the doctor owns the hospital.

Mixed systems

Some countries use a mix of systems. For example, certain clear cut diagnoses are paid on a lump-sum basis (common operations and deliveries) while for other diagnoses the payment is per day with an extra payment for three categories of operation – major, medium and minor. As mentioned earlier, prior approval may be required for further days of stay beyond a quota given on admission according to diagnosis.

Conclusion on paying hospitals

There is no perfect way of paying a hospital. Any method will create some perverse incentives. Each country must choose whatever system is least likely to be abused, given the pattern of ownership of the hospitals concerned, the effectiveness of any inspection or accreditation system, and the ethical standards of those concerned.

The pharmacist

It is generally the practice in Europe for private pharmacists to dispense prescriptions written by doctors working outside hospitals. The prices of the drugs sold to the pharmacist in bulk are regulated and the permitted mark up of the pharmacist is negotiated. If this is a percentage of the cost, the pharmacists have an incentive to dispense the more expensive brands where they have discretion to do so. A flat-rate dispensing fee does not have this effect. Nor does payment on a capitation basis, as is being tried out in the Netherlands. This, of course, means that the patient has to register with one pharmacy. Another way of encouraging pharmacists to select a cheaper product where they have a choice is used in Western Germany. The insurer fixes the maximum which it will pay for each range of similar products – a 'reference price'. The pharmacists then know that they will have to charge the patient any extra cost. This system is being copied in the Netherlands and Denmark.

The pharmacist sends prescriptions each month to the insurer who prices them and pays the pharmacist. This enables the insurer to see that only those drugs permitted under the regulations are prescribed and to keep computer records of the prescribing of each doctor and use them to inform each doctor of his or her prescribing pattern and apply sanctions in cases of excessive prescribing.

Conclusion

As shown above, every system of securing the payment of providers has potential disadvantages. There is no right answer. All of them can, however, be made to work. Ways have been found of overcoming the worst disadvantages of nearly all systems. But some of them are costly to operate and what would be tolerated by providers in one country may be opposed to the point of strike action in another. This is why each country must work out what would suit it best. In choosing between ways of paying providers, the administrative cost of different systems should not be overlooked. The aim is not to minimise such costs but to secure that such costs are balanced against the gains in efficiency, economy and the acceptability of services to users which can be generated by them.

Notes

1 Patag, F. (1983), *Medical care system in the Philippines, ASIA/RT/SEO, ISSA.*
2 Glaser, W.A. (1991), *Health Insurance in Practice*, Jossey-Bass, San Francisco.

3 Abel-Smith, B. and Grandjeat, P. (1978), *Pharmaceutical Consumption*, Commission of the European Communities, Brussels.
4 McPherson, K. *et al.* (1978), 'Regional variations in the use of common surgical procedures', *Social Science and Medicine*, vol. 15A.
5 Kim, Y.J. (1987), 'Health care financing in Korea', Seminar on Health Care Financing, Asian Development Bank, (unpublished).
6 Beech, R. and Morgan M. (1992), 'Constraints on innovatory practice: The case of day surgery in the NHS', *International Journal of Health Planning and Management*, vol. 7.

CHAPTER 15

The efficient use of health resources

Efficiency has a number of aspects. Two important ones are technical efficiency and consumer acceptability. The first is concerned with whether necessary and quality care was provided at the lowest cost? Consumer acceptability is concerned with user satisfaction. For example, is the care which users receive prompt, acceptable and courteous. Are they kept fully informed and their dignity respected? Are visitors made welcome? This depends partly on training and supervision but also on how providers are paid, as pointed out in the last chapter. But it also depends on whether the patient can choose, so that there is competition between providers and money follows the patient.

Technical efficiency

The possible ways of increasing technical efficiency are legion. One is by securing the rational use of essential drugs, as discussed in chapter 9. A second is by changing the incentives operating on providers through payment systems, as discussed in chapter 14. A third is by the careful planning of the quantity, type and location of hospitals, as discussed in chapter 10. A fourth is by careful reviews of staffing levels against work loads and the use of expensive resources.

The key to finding possible gains in efficiency is information about what is really going on in the health services. In developed countries the key problems are unnecessary admissions to hospital, excessive lengths of stay, excessive use of diagnostic tests, irrational prescribing and over-prescribing. The same problems are found in some developing countries, particularly in Eastern Europe and China. Irrational prescribing is a world problem. In both developed and developing countries, there is the additional problem of unnecessary care. It has been estimated that 10–30 per cent of the actions performed at the secondary and tertiary level in Latin America are absolutely unnecessary. Examples include caesarean section rates of 50 per cent or higher, unnecessarily high rates of elective surgery and excessive use of laboratory services and X-rays (Banta 1988: p. 16)[1]. The WHO Regional Committee for the Americas estimated that possibly some 30 per cent of the total resources available to the health sector in the Latin American countries were lost through wastage, for such reasons as the inadequacy of technology and deficiencies in management (WHO 1985: p. 13)[2]. No estimates are available for developing countries in Asia or Africa.

Problems can be identified by comparisons between the performance of different clinicians, hospitals, areas, provinces and countries. In most countries, a large amount of prescribed drugs are wasted because the patient does not take them as directed. Administrators hesitate to act directly on these problems because to do so would challenge professional freedom and other vested interests. There are, however, ways of acting indirectly such as, for example, imposing budgets, and using a variety of systems of regulation as discussed in chapter 11 and changing the incentives operating on providers.

In many of the poorer developing countries, the information system is inadequate or not functioning as intended due to the fall in morale of health service staffs and difficulties in communication between the different levels of the health system, which may in part be due to the lack of functioning vehicles and the lack of fuel. Without even the basic information about the activity of the health services, such as curative and preventive visits, admissions and lengths of stay and even the deployment of personnel, it is not possible to attempt the most obvious task of seeing whether staff are being used in the most efficient way. Thus there are often health centres with more staff than they need for their tasks, who idle away the day or cultivate their private plots for half the day, while other health units are seriously over-stretched and cannot do anything like all that is expected of them. Similarly nurses and doctors are not fairly distributed between hospitals.

The second problem is that the existing information systems were seldom designed to give the information that management would need in order to assess efficiency. It is seldom that there is systematic information about functioning equipment. Thus equipment in one health unit lies idle awaiting repair, while in another unit there may be functioning equipment but a lack of staff who can use it. A study in Colombia looked in 1982 at all the 1,289 pieces of medical equipment provided under the European aid programmes from 1974 to 1979 and found that 95 per cent was not functioning (WHO 1985: p. 23)[3].

But the largest failing is the lack of any system of costing which could be used for management. Many ex-colonies have retained the old-fashioned type of line budgeting system which only shows the type of goods and services used, but cannot be broken down into the health units using them. A system of this kind has two intrinsic faults. First, the hospital directors cannot switch resources between alternative uses without the clumsy process of asking for permission. Thus costly and inconvenient delays in the care of patients may arise while permission is sought. Second, it is not possible to find out the costs of different health units to compare with units of activity. The stocks have come and gone from central medical stores but to which unit they went has not been recorded. Indeed many supplies may have 'fallen off the back of the lorry' into the black market. With the collapse of supervision there has often also been a collapse of local auditing. No one, for example, compares drugs supplied with drugs listed in the day book as prescribed, quite apart from advising on rational prescribing. And even if these records are properly kept, there may be no record of whether they were actually supplied. This is an invitation to theft.

As pointed out in chapter 10, one of the most glaring inequities is in the large tertiary hospitals. The difficulties of seriously ill patients taking up referrals, because of lack of transport throughout the health services, coupled with lack of public transport (if the patient could use it), often means that most of the work of a tertiary hospital is the same as that done in a district hospital or a primary health care unit but at much higher cost.

Even if the requisite information were available, ministries of health usually lack the staff to draw the correct conclusions from it. Usually, a weighting system has to be developed to compare costs fairly between different health units for different activities (such as the case mix or inpatient versus outpatient work of hospitals). Specialised staff are needed to select the areas which most need further investigation for action by senior management. Very few ministries have trained health economists and, if they have, there is a reluctance to allow them to challenge the inherited wisdom of the medical planners. Finally, there may be a reluctance to disturb the status quo for political reasons. Thus it is better not to know.

This is, of course, not true of health services in all developing countries. Some ministries do a remarkably good job in these respects and some are developing management information systems to do so (e.g. Thailand). But most have one or more of the failings mentioned above. The savings in the better use of resources could undoubtedly be large.

Technology

As pointed out in chapter 11, technological innovation is the largest single cause of the increase in the cost of health services in developed countries. It is also of great importance in developing countries. Rising cost is not so much due to greater use of technology, but because more expensive technologies are constantly replacing or more often supplementing cheaper ones. Thus securing that the technology used is appropriate and necessary needs to play an important part in securing efficiency in the use of health service resources.

What is appropriate in one context may not be in another. To become reliant on a technology which needs regular maintenance by highly skilled technicians, where such technicians are not available, is clearly inappropriate. Similarly, to depend on electricity when the supply is irregular and of varying voltage is inappropriate where alternatives are available. For example, coal or wood can be used for boiling water and, if properly maintained, the temperature can be kept consistently low in a paraffin refrigerator: in the long run solar-powered refrigerators may become affordable. A water pump which local people can maintain is to be preferred to a model with higher power which needs skilled maintenance.

In its broadest sense technology can be defined as the 'equipment, devices, drugs and procedures employed in the care of patients . . . including capital and human investment' (Fineberg and Hiatt 1979: pp. 1086–91)[4]. But the major concern is expensive medical technology. A technology can fall into this category either because it involves expensive capital equipment (e.g. a whole body scanner), or because it requires substantial time of highly skilled persons to operate it (e.g. renal dialysis) or because of high utilisation (e.g. diagnostic tests or certain drugs) (Balaban and Goldfarb 1988: p. 17)[5]. It has been found, for example, in the United States that age- and sex-adjusted surgical rates for such common procedures as tonsillectomy, hysterectomy and open heart surgery are six times higher in the highest region than in the lowest without any discernible difference in health status before or after.

Abandoned technologies

It is much easier to show that technologies have been inappropriately used in the past than to prove that newer or retained technologies are inappropriate. This is partly because of the difficulties of measuring the benefits of a technology, partly because of the powerful placebo effect which has been often measured (Skrabanek and McCormick 1989: pp. 6–19)[6] and partly because of the ethical problems of attempting to do so, once a technology has been elevated into the position of the 'preferred treatment'.

The history of discarded technologies is long and sad. By the mid 1930s, X-rays of the foetus had become routine: they were abandoned once it was found that they could cause leukaemia (Oakley 1984: pp. 102–5)[7]. Cancer patients were treated with vitamin C until it was found it did no good and might be harmful (Skrabanek and McCormick 1989: p. 36)[8]. In the past patients with myocardial infarcts were ordered to bed for six weeks and some developed clots in their legs as a result. Now early mobilisation within 24 hours is the rule (Skrabanek and McCormick 1989: p. 37)[9]. Gastric freezing was rapidly adopted and equally rapidly abandoned. Amniocentesis was widely used before it was known that it could damage the foetus, when its use became confined to cases where a blood test indicated a higher than average risk of abnormality and abortion was acceptable to the parents. A high concentration of oxygen was used for premature babies until it was found to be associated with the development of retrolental fibroplasia (Silverman 1980)[10]. Full mastectomy was the most common treatment for cancer of the breast, until it became known that similar results could be obtained by small local operations. Tonsillectomies were frequently used, with some risk of mortality from the anaesthetic, until it was appreciated that most cases recover without treatment.

More common is the overuse of technologies when there is no clear benefit from their use. Electronic fetal monitoring is still often used for pregnant women although a trial showed no benefit (Williams 1982: p. 38)[11]. Cervical screening was widely used long before it was known how often to use it or what age and socio-economic groups were most at risk. Once electro-convulsive therapy was found to be beneficial for depression it was widely used for other mental illnesses. Coronary care units were widely used before it was known what indications justified their use. Special care units were introduced for low weight babies – about 6 per cent of births – but became used for 17 per cent by 1977 by adding malformed babies and also forceps or caesarean deliveries, despite the damage to the bonding of mother and child. In the case of newer technologies, it is still not known in what cases the use of CAT scanners or ultrasonic scanners leads to a reduction of morbidity or mortality.

The problem is that a doctor of high reputation reports good results from a new treatment in a journal, often from only a small number of cases. Others follow and report similar good results and it does not take long before it becomes the preferred treatment for the whole flock of the profession. What is not clear is whether the good results were due to the treatment or the confidence of the patients in their doctors – the placebo effect.

Evaluating technologies

Research that proves that a treatment is beneficial is difficult at any time and likely to be resisted on ethical grounds once a treatment is widely adopted. Before and after studies may not give reliable results because of the placebo effect. Matched control groups are always at risk of the matching being imperfect in some respect. Thus a random control trial in which patients are allocated at random to the new treatment and to no treatment or to the old treatment can provide hard evidence. Ideally neither the doctor nor the patient should know what treatment (e.g. a drug) is being given – a 'double blind trial'. But in the case of most treatments the doctor has to know how to administer it, introducing again some risk of a placebo effect – a 'single blind trial'.

For a random control trial to be undertaken, those with the skills to organise it need to get in early, but often they do not hear about the new development in time. Technologies often slip into use without needing new equipment or, if they do, with equipment loaned or sold at a discount by the manufacturer. And by no means all clinicians are prepared to cooperate with a trial. The attempt to establish one, by authorising equipment only for qualified research centres on condition that a trial is launched, can be frustrated if donors are found to pay for equipment for other units before the results of the trial are available.

Three questions need answering (White 1982: pp. 10–12)[12]. The first is whether the technology does what it claims to do. The results of the test need to be valid, accurate and reliable in the sense that they are reproducible by other observers. The second question is whether it is effective and for which patients. Does it reduce mortality, morbidity, disability, discomfort or dissatisfaction in the patient? The third question is whether it is efficient. What gain is achieved at what cost and to whom? These last two questions raise difficult problems of values. Who is to assess the improvement and how is it to be measured – the doctor, the patient or the patient's relatives?

The important point is that very few technologies have been fully evaluated. Sir Douglas Black estimated that only 10 per cent of diseases are significantly influenced by modern treatment (Black 1984)[13]. A recent committee set up by the government of the Netherlands concluded that 'medical technology, mainly devices and their application, be subjected to the same requirements of effectiveness and safety as are drugs, before being approved for health care' (Ministry of Welfare 1992: p. 134)[14]. The task was to be done by an independent agency. But this does not deal with existing technologies.

Developing countries can least afford the use of ineffective technologies or the overuse of effective technologies where they are not effective. Where their resources only allow one or two machines to be bought, there are opportunities for random control trials which are no longer available in countries where all have access to the technology. This is simply because the limited resources make it inevitable that the majority of patients will be denied the use of the technology whether there is a trial or not. The argument that a trial would be unethical cannot be maintained. The developed countries would have a clear interest in offering financial and other support for such trials but it is important that there are proper ethical safeguards.

But the important responsibility rests with developed countries not to allow the introduction of further new and expensive technologies without proper evaluation. There are signs that at least some countries (such as the Netherlands and Denmark) are beginning to try to accept this responsibility. How successful they will be remains to be seen.

The role of the private sector

The private sector of health services plays a considerable role in the health systems of both developed and developing countries. The role is generally larger in the latter, though its quantitative role is seldom fully documented. The private sector has been defined to cover both for-profit private companies and individuals, and not-for-profit private organisations (non-governmental organisations) and include all those organisations and individuals working outside the direct control of the state (Bennett 1991: p. 4)[15].

In many countries polarised attitudes are taken to the role of the private sector. In some countries, the private sector is regarded by the public sector as a dangerous predator, robbing the public sector of trained workers, particularly nurses, and distracting doctors by its higher earnings from their main work which ought to be in the public sector. If only government was in a position to give the public sector enough resources, there would be no need for the private sector to exist, except in a very minor role. Others regard the private sector as the long-term answer to the provision of health care, as public services are bound to be inefficient, bureaucratic and impersonal. Because the private sector has to respond to market forces, this is bound to make it both efficient and user-friendly. The World Bank argued in 1987 that an expanded role for markets and the private sector increases both allocative and technical efficiency in the financing and provision of services (World Bank 1987)[16]. Some bank officials have even argued that public hospitals or health centres should be handed over or sold to the private sector, or failing that, profit-making management companies should be brought in to run them.

Privatisation

The slogan for those who would wish blindly to increase the role of the private sector is 'privatisation'. Yet this term is used to cover two quite different issues – transferring production from the public sector to the private sector and transferring costs from the public sector to the private sector. The latter was discussed in chapter 12 above. Here we are only concerned with the transfer of production. The provision of health services cannot simply be handed over to the private sector because of the substantial imperfections of the health market. As the World Bank put it, two years later, in a more cautious mood, 'a private market can operate efficiently only if it works within the environment of a well-functioning market system, which provides price signals that accurately reflect the social and financial costs of production' (World Bank 1989)[17]. Because of the ignorance of consumers about what treatment they need and all the uncertainties and problems of equity, the price signals do not reflect the social and financial costs of production. Nor is changing ownership a panacea. Competitiveness is more important than ownership in stimulating efficiency. Private ownership by no means implies competitiveness and it may be possible to stimulate competitive conditions within the public sector. 'Economic theory is not able to give a clear-cut answer to the appropriate mix between public and private sectors. This must be decided on a case by case basis' (Bennett 1991: p. 21)[18]. In particular, factors such as the characteristics of the current health system and existing socio-economic conditions must be taken into account, as these determine the feasibility of potential changes in the mix.

Thus it is argued that 'attempts at privatisation are likely to encounter serious difficulties unless consideration has also been given to the development of appropriate incentive structures and ways to control costs, retain manpower and ensure satisfactory quality in the private sector' (Bennett 1991: p. 45)[19]. In other words, enhancing the role of the private sector requires a strengthened and expanded role for government.

This does not lend support to those who would wish to see the private sector wither away. But the important point is that enhancing the role of the private sector should be approached empirically with understanding of the actual situation in a particular country.

One important area where valuable progress has been made in many developing countries is the training of traditional practitioners and birth attendants. The public sector is very unlikely to be able to compete with them in accessibility, acceptability and convenience.

He does not try to put you in hospital far from friends and relatives, among apparently uninterested doctors and nurses, where, as like as not, you will run into difficulties with the disposal of lochia or faeces, or where you will be given food which you know is harmful. Neither does he laugh at you when you ascribe your disease to a punishment for some emotion or to magic. He gives treatment with his own hand and does not send you to a pharmacist, nor ask payment of you in advance of results. He does not reveal his ignorance by asking questions or requiring elaborate tests. He does not take notes which may have a magical hold on you. He never says he does not know what is the matter with you. (Brockington 1985: p. 124)

The services of traditional practitioners are attuned to the culture, and traditional birth attendants are generally willing to give much wider services than a trained midwife, including care of other children, cooking and cleaning. Teaching traditional practitioners how to use a limited range of Western drugs enhances their prestige and traditional birth attendants can be issued with equipment which is easy to clean, and they have been successfully used to impress on mothers the importance of immunisation and to make them aware of the availability of family planning services.

A second area is to contract out the cleaning, laundry and catering services of hospitals. The practicability of this depends on the availability of enough local firms to compete for the contracts which may not exist in some developing countries. It also depends on the competence of hospital managements in specifying the requirements under the contract in detail and constantly monitoring the observance of its terms (Bennett 1991: pp. 32–33)[21]. Bids by outside contractors should be compared with the cost of continuing to use directly employed labour.

A third area, often suggested for privatisation, is medical education. Why not take the load off government by encouraging private self-financing medical schools, provided the standard of their examination is ratified by some central agency? The case against is that a medical school driven by market forces will very likely try to become a preparatory school for training in specialties. For these reasons, it is argued that the government cannot afford to relinquish direct control of the medical curriculum. On the other hand there may well be a role for privatisation in the alternative sense of increasing private funding. It is hard to justify free medical education being provided at public expense to the children of rich families. There is a strong case for parents paying according to their means with scholarships established only for those children from poorer families who meet the admission requirements.

Another area to approach with caution and careful empirical investigation is the transfer of public health services (health centres and hospitals) to non-governmental organisations or profit-making companies operating with a government subsidy or under contract with the government. Private profit-making hospitals do not necessarily give better value for money. A careful comparison by the Institute of Medicine in the United States came to the conclusion that the ability of profit-making hospitals to produce the same services at lower cost had not been demonstrated (Institute of Medicine 1986)[22]. Similarly, bringing in private firms to manage non-profit hospitals, which was the fashion from the 1970s, did not result in savings in costs. The situation of the United States is, of course, very different from that typically found in developing countries. Virtually all hospitals in the United States employ professionally trained managers. This is rarely the case in public hospitals in developing countries where management is generally in the hands of a senior clinician who has been given no specific training for the job. An additional liability is the absence of a hospital costing system. Often the manager does not have in practice the right to dismiss unsatisfactory staff either for political reasons or because the procedures for doing so are too protracted to make it worth initiating them.

In these circumstances, it is more likely to be the case that profit-making hospitals or not-for-profit hospitals, both of which have at least to cover their costs, are run more efficiently. They need to have a costing system to stay in business. It is commonly believed that mission hospitals provide quality care efficiently but there is only limited data to support this (Bennett 1991: p. 35)[23]. For-profit hospitals may, on the other hand, be subject to quite different types of pressure leading to inefficiency. If the doctors, ultimately responsible for the care of the patients, are charging the patients on a fee-for-service basis, they are tempted to order unnecessary tests and do unnecessary procedures for which both the hospital and the doctor can charge the patient. Secondly, they may need to provide patients with a much higher standard of amenity than could be afforded in a public hospital. This is necessary to attract patients to pay to use them. In other words, they are geared to serve much higher income groups than the public hospitals.

These complications make it very difficult to make fair comparisons of costs. But at the initial stage of making comparisons, public hospitals need to establish a costing system and that system must be able to get down to the detail of costing different types of case. This is essential for making any fair comparisons. One reason why private hospitals may appear to give greater value for money may be because they select their cases carefully – avoiding those that require complex or prolonged care, which are left to the public sector.

A further important point is that of quality. The ambivalent, if not hostile, attitude to the private sector by the public sector often leads to grossly inadequate procedures to safeguard the quality of care given in private hospitals. It is commonly the case that private hospitals, once licensed, are never subject to further inspection unless there are complaints. The initial licensing may have been based simply on the suitability of the building from a public health point of view – covering such questions as water, sanitation, lighting, ventilation, bed-spacing and the safe storage of dangerous drugs. In many cases the legislation governing registration has been left unrevised for many years and the suitability of the building may have deteriorated since approval was given using these minimal criteria.

An effective system of quality control needs at the least to cover the ratios of qualified staff to beds (on duty both by day and night), the availability of functioning equipment, the question of which doctors are able to attempt what surgery and the provision of qualified staff to provide anaesthetics. Moreover any standards need to be enforced by regular visits of which no notice is given. The easiest way for a hospital to economise and add to its profits is by the dilution of the quality of its staff. Patients rarely enquire what qualifications are possessed by persons dressed in white coats when they are described as 'nurses'!

Thus it is extremely dangerous for an incoming minister, with a dogmatic approach to privatisation, to imagine that he or she can solve the problem of inefficiencies in the public sector by waving this magic wand. What would be useful would be to take the initial steps of removing obstacles which obstruct the ability of public sector managers to manage, introducing hospital costing, sending existing public hospital managers for training and establishing much more thorough courses to develop the hospital managers of the future. There is no reason why these managers should be doctors. They generally are not, either in the United States or in many countries in Western Europe. Similarly an effective system of quality assurance needs to be established for private hospitals.

Encouraging competition

As pointed out above, competition is much more important than ownership in creating efficiency. How far is it possible to establish effective competition in the health sector – between public sector health units as well as between units in the public and private sectors? This raises the further questions of who should decide to distribute custom between competing contractors – the patient or some intermediate agency – and whether there should be limits to choice.

Competition in health care is by no means a new idea, though it has been given revived popularity in the writings of Alain Enthoven in the United States (Enthoven 1988: pp. 305–21)[24]. Nor is what the Americans now call 'managed care'. By 1900, the German sick funds operating compulsory health insurance were selecting those doctors who gave a service which was both economical and of an acceptable quality. They monitored each doctor's use of resources. They used what the Americans now call 'preferred providers'. Similarly the British sick funds, before national health insurance, selected their doctors on the basis of quality and price. These arrangements were not popular with those doctors who were excluded in either country and it was the government in both cases that finally gave all doctors the right to participate in compulsory health insurance, thereby removing competition by price and quality (Abel-Smith 1988)[25]. In Germany, the choice included both specialists and general practitioners. In the United Kingdom choice was limited to general practitioners in the first instance: specialists could only be seen on referral. This last restriction of choice is cost-effective, as pointed out in chapter 14.

Competition between, and within, public and private hospitals has, however, continued right up to the present in such countries as Belgium, France, Germany and the Netherlands and there are no plans to abolish it. Money follows the patients' choices. Hospitals which are not popular with patients will lose custom and, therefore, money and hospitals which are popular gain both. Competition makes all hospitals attempt to be user-friendly.

The British reform

It was the principle of competition which Mrs Thatcher decided to extend to the British National Health Service. What worried her was that she found herself driven to spend more and more on the health service despite what she saw as its evident inefficiencies – large variations in inpatient costs, waiting lists, doctors' prescribing habits and particularly in referral rates to specialists (UK Government 1989: p. 3)[26].

Her aim was to make the health service buy its services taking account of quality and price to make it cost conscious on private sector management principles. She also wanted to increase the freedom of local managers to manage: the larger public hospitals were freed from the main rules of the National Health Service and, for example, were allowed to determine the pay of their employees rather than observe nationally negotiated pay scales, while still being publicly owned.

The reform, introduced in 1991, was based on a simple proposition. While consumers can judge a user-friendly service, they cannot judge quality nor, in a largely free service, can they be expected to care about price. Thus an intermediary needs to be brought in to do the buying of hospital and specialist services, who is more skilled in judging quality and does care about price. Two intermediaries are being used. First are the larger general practices. They are given budgets with which to buy many of the specialist and hospital services which they need for their patients. In the long run these budgets will be based on the number of patients each practice is looking after – a capitation basis – probably with an adjustment for the age of the patient. The incentive is that any profit made on the annual budget can be spent on improving the practice. A proposal for Spain went further and suggested that the doctors could put the profit in their pockets.

The more innovative family doctor practices are already showing their teeth (Glennerster *et al.* 1992)[27]. Their contracts with hospitals may, for example:

- specify the times within which an appointment should be made, require the dates of appointments to be sent to the practice by fax and that patients should be seen within specified time limits after arrival and by a consultant, not a junior doctor, on the first visit unless there are exceptional circumstances;
- decide to refer their patients where they can be seen more quickly;
- require consultants to give their outpatient service in the GP's own surgery;
- insist on their permission being obtained for further outpatient visits after the first one or two.
- require laboratory tests results to be returned on the same day by courier instead of receiving a weekly service from the hospital.

Oddly enough the fund-holding model was also one of the reforms introduced in the Soviet Union during the period of the Gorbachev reforms. There it was called 'the Leningrad experiment'. This is one of the models now being used in Sweden. Nigeria is planning a similar model under the new insurance scheme which it is hoped soon to introduce.

The second purchaser is the district management which is now told to contract with hospitals, public and private, on the basis of price and quality. This acts for the smaller general practices or those that are currently not equipped or are unwilling to take the risk of becoming fund-holders. Thus the district management has changed its role from controlling hospitals to contracting them. A similar system is planned to be introduced by the new democratic government in Chile throughout its public hospital services. And the reform introduced in New Zealand in 1993 entirely separates the agency to do the buying from the agency that controls the services.

There are five main difficulties in the British reform. The first is whether it is possible for quality to be measured and thus become a serious consideration in the placing and monitoring of contracts. The second is to assemble reliable costing information for each hospital. The third is how to prevent the larger general practices from selecting low health-risk patients. The fourth is to prevent general practitioners from attempting tasks which are beyond their competence because they lack recent experience of them. The fifth is the risk that patients who are not in fund-holding practices will get poorer services than those who are. Countries considering the possibility of introducing this approach need to appreciate that, to work effectively, it requires a very high standard of managerial competence.

The Dutch reform

The reform in the Netherlands is rather different (Wynand 1988)[28]. There have long been a variety of different insurers most of them operating on a non-profit basis. The central aim is to achieve the efficient use of resources by creating price competition between insurers, by the latter in turn creating competition between providers and by integrating the financing of each insured person's health and social care.

Under the plan, the whole population would be compulsorily insured for what are called 'basic health services' – hospital specialist, nursing home and other health care at present provided by the social welfare services. Each individual would have the right to choose an insurer and insurers would not be allowed to refuse to accept a customer or adjust premiums to risk. About 93 per cent of the cost of the insurance would be paid from compulsory contributions charged at standard rates related to income. Children would be covered by their parents' contributions. This contribution would be collected centrally and distributed between insurers on a capitation basis – according to the number of insured persons and their risk status (age would be one variable). The rest of the contribution would fall on the individual as a flat-rate payment and would vary according to the chosen insurer but each insurer would have to charge the same premium to all its insured persons. Each insurer would be free to negotiate prices with hospitals.

Thus insurers become intermediaries between the consumer and the provider seeking to buy acceptable and quality hospital care at a favourable price. Insurers would be free to restrict the providers which their insured persons are allowed to use. Insurers must accept people on first entering insurance and changing from another insurer.

Thus the scheme gives the consumer choice of insurer and is intended to encourage a variety of contracting arrangements with hospitals from which the consumer can choose. The scheme creates competition between providers as each insurer is negotiating separately instead of each insurer having to accept, as previously, the price and type of contract negotiated centrally by the association of insurers. Thus insurers have incentives to see that less costly alternatives to care in hospital are fully exploited when they can provide satisfactory care.

Wider uses for capitation

One common feature of these reforms is the use of the capitation basis for distributing money between those responsible for contracting. Capitation is a very flexible instrument and can be used in a variety of ways as is shown by recent changes in developing countries. For example in Bali (Indonesia), family doctors are given capitation payments out of which they not only have to provide their own services but the drugs they prescribe for their patients as well. This is a way of encouraging economical prescribing which was long used under voluntary insurance in Europe in the nineteenth century.

Under the new Thailand health insurance scheme, those who are insured make a choice of hospital. This hospital then receives a capitation payment for each insured person who chooses it. The hospital is then expected to make two further types of contract: with a tertiary hospital ('super-contractors') for cases which it refers to it and pays it for its services; and with primary care providers (sub-contactors) which it can pay mainly on a capitation basis but possibly supplemented by fees for defined preventive services. The advantage of this model is the decentralisation of so much of the contracting process which gives local flexibility. It can be introduced quicker than many of the other models, because of the decentralisation of responsibility and the avoidance of the complex problem of finding a way to pay hospitals on the basis of the cases they treat which would take substantial time to develop.

Conclusion

Thus the message that it is competition that matters rather than ownership is beginning to spread around the world. But the task of changing over to a competitive system should not be underestimated. Competition cannot operate on the basis of costs until costs are known. For many countries, collecting this information will be a major undertaking. It may seem that reintroducing some of the magic of market functioning can solve all the problems of efficiency. There is no doubt that these mechanisms could get services at low cost. However the process of contracting is by no means costless for the contractor or for the body placing the contract. But the major problems with these models is how to build in guarantees of quality and prevent discrimination against high health-risk users.

Notes

1   Banta, H.D. (1988), 'The transfer of medical technologies in developing countries' in Rutten, F.F.H. and Reiser, S.J. (eds.), *The Economics of Medical Technology*, Springer-Verlag, Berlin.
2   World Health Organisation (1985), 'Planning of the finances for Health for All', (-E77/INF.DOC/1) WHO (unpublished).
3   WHO (1985), 'Planning of the finances'
4   Fineberg, H.V. and Hiatt, H.H. (1979), 'Evaluation of medical practices: the cases for technology assessment', *New England Journal of Medicine*, vol. 301, no. 20.
5   Balaban, D.J. and Goldfarb, N.I. (1982), 'Medical evaluation of health care technologies' in Culyer, A.J. and Horisberger, B. (eds.) *Economic and Medical Evaluation of Health Care Technologies*, Springer-Verlag, Berlin.
6   Skrabanek, P. and McCormick, J. (1989), *Follies and Fallacies in Medicine*, Tarragon, Glasgow.
7   Oakley, A. (1984), *The Captured Womb*, Blackwell, Oxford.
8   Skrabanek and McCormick (1989), *Follies and Fallacies*.
9   Skrabanek and McCormick (1989), *Follies and Fallacies*.
10 Silverman, W.A. (1980), *Retrolental Fibroplasia – a Modern Parable*, Monographs in Neonatology, Grune and Stratton, New York.
11 Williams, A. (1982), 'The role of economics in the evaluation of health care technologies', in Culyer, A.J. and Horisberger, B. (eds.) *Economic and Medical Evaluation*.
12 White, K.L. (1982), 'Evaluation and medicine', in Culyer, A.J. and Horisberger, B. (eds.), *Economic and Medical Evaluation*.
13 Black, D. (1984), *An Anthology of False Antitheses*, Nuffield Provincial Trust, London.
14 Ministry of Welfare, Health and Cultural Affairs (1992), *Choices in Health Care*, Government of the Netherlands, Rijswijk.
15 Bennett, S. (1991), *The Mystique of Markets: Public and Private Health Care in Developing Countries*, PHP Departmental Publications No. 4, London School of Hygiene and Tropical Medicine, London.
16 World Bank (1987), *Financing Health Services in Developing Countries; an Agenda for Reform*, World Bank, Washington D.C.
17 World Bank (1989), *Developing the Private Sector: a Challenge for the World Bank Group*, World Bank, Washington D.C.
18 Bennett (1991), *The Mystique of Markets*.

19   Bennett (1991), *The Mystique of Markets*.
20   Brockington, F. (1985), *The Health of the Developing World*, Book Guild, Lewes.
21   Bennett (1991), *The Mystique of Markets*.
22   Institute of Medicine (1986), *For Profit Enterprise in Health Care*, National Academy Press, Washington D.C.
23   Bennett (1991), *The Mystique of Markets*.
24   Enthoven, A.C. (1988), 'Managed competition of alternative delivery systems', *Journal of Health Politics, Policy and Law*, vol. 13, no. 2.
25   Abel-Smith, B. (1988), 'The Rise and decline of the early HMOs: some international experiences', *Milbank Quarterly*, vol. 66, no. 4.
26   UK Government (1989), *Working for Patients*, HMSO, London.
27   Glennerster, H. *et al.* (1992), *A Foothold for Fundholding*, King's Fund Institute, London.
28   Wynand, P.M.M. van der Ven (1988), *A Future for Competitive Health Care in the Netherlands*, Occasional Paper No. 9, Centre for Health Economics, York.

CHAPTER 16

Facing up to the future

This final chapter, at the cost of some repetition, sums up the main themes of this book. No country can meet all possible demands for health services. Therefore health planning should start from what is affordable and will be affordable in the future.

In the past, health plans have been based only on short-term considerations. Often they have consisted only of plans for capital developments. Some plans in developing countries have amounted to little more than shopping lists presented hopefully to donors. But in so far as they involve capital developments, whether in the form of hospitals, equipment or the training of further personnel, what is critical is the increase in recurrent costs which are likely to be generated which will have to be met from national resources. It is no use being absurdly optimistic about the future. In the few cases where forward plans have been costed, it is not unknown to show very modest increases in expenditure for the next few years, followed by quite disproportionate increases in expenditure in later years. They represent bids for funds rather than cool assessments of the funds likely to be made available.

Major problems have been created by the failure to look ahead and face up to the long-term consequences of short-term decisions. Training schools have been established, particularly for doctors without thought of whether the money will be available either from the public sector or the private sector to provide a living for the health professionals once they have been trained. Work-force plans have often been simply 'needs-based' representing what it is hoped to be able to afford, not what is likely to be affordable. Hospitals have been built in developing countries, often with donor support, without even calculating their future running costs, let alone seeing whether it is likely to be possible to contain these running costs within future health budgets. By no means all the problems now facing so many developing countries were created by the economic crisis. Some would have faced severe problems of finding recurrent resources even if health budgets had continued at the level existing before the economic crisis.

Many health ministries in developing countries are so overcome by the problems of trying to maintain some credible health service on the resources currently available that their overwhelming task is living from day to day and trying to manage one crisis after another. Will there be a strike if the payment of health staff is delayed because of inadequate resources? What is the fairest way of distributing grossly inadequate funds for drugs, let alone petrol or vehicle maintenance? Is it possible politically to delay the opening of the new hospital, the construction of which played some part in getting the current government elected? Is it less damaging to the government to cut grants to non-governmental organisations which have long been providing the main services in some areas than to admit that government hospitals will have to be seriously under-financed? Are protests more likely if urban facilities are starved of resources than if the rural areas are made to go short? The author has visited countries where each of these questions has been asked and answered.

Making a financial plan

In the current situation it may seem unrealistic to suggest that all countries should plan for the future, particularly as the experience of the past decade has suggested that so many important determinants of the economic situation can change and change rapidly in ways which could not have been predicted. The fact that the future is so uncertain is not a reason for making no plans. But it is a reason for making plans which verge on the side of pessimism – that assume that things are unlikely to get better and may even get worse. Cutting, in the short period, the consequences of an over-ambitious plan is much more difficult, as many countries have been learning to their cost, than adding to a modest plan if the economic prospects become better than previously assumed. A plan can be based on alternative scenarios from very pessimistic to modestly optimistic. At least this will help to identify the key issues at stake.

The content of a plan

A plan sets out what will be provided in the future – what buildings, personnel and supplies. Critically, it takes account of capital developments – construction costs followed by the running costs which will follow from the construction of new buildings or the rehabilitation of existing buildings, and investments in training programmes followed by provision for the payment of those who have been trained. The centre point of a plan is long-term running costs and what level of finance might be available and what could be accommodated within that level of finance. If not, are there ways of augmenting the finance likely to be available from existing policies? A plan forces countries to face up to what may and what may not be affordable under differing economic conditions. This gives messages for current decision-making – particularly not to plan for the unaffordable. Thus the primary challenge is to plan 'Health for All' within realistic estimates of resources which can be made available from all possible sources of finance. The secondary challenge is to stretch the resources which can be made available by an imaginative and bold search for ways to increase efficiency.

In WHO's original specifications for 'Health for All', it was agreed that there would be global plans or strategies, followed by regional plans or strategies. There would then be global and regional indicators and a plan for research. These stages have been completed. The next stage was intended to be national plans. They were to start with a national strategy statement, and many countries have got as far as this step. Next there were to be financial plans, plans for personnel and a detailed plan of action (see Table 16.1). Few countries have followed through to these later stages.

Table 16.1   **The process of Health for All planning (as recommended by WHO)**

GLOBAL AND REGIONAL
Strategy
Indicators
Research Programme
Monitoring
Evaluation

NATIONAL
Strategy
Financial Plan
Work-force Plan
Construction Plan
Plan of action

In terms of the programme budgeting set out in chapter 6 above, long-term financial planning was a component of the second stage – broad programming. It tests the financial feasibility of the whole of the proposed programme. Implementation is through detailed programming with finance provided through the annual budget process.

The financial plan was intended to cover all health expenditures and how they were financed:

- for health-related activity as well as health services;
- for capital and current expenditure separately;
- for the private sector as well as the public sector (including the relevant activities of all government departments and compulsory social security institutions);
- for training as well as services and other activities;
- for regional as well as national activities;
- for primary care as well as secondary care.

The uncertainties about the future were only one reason for the failure to make financial plans. Other reasons include the lack of competence in ministries of health for undertaking such an unfamiliar task, which required some basic knowledge of the simpler economic concepts. While the economic planners have the skills in macro-planning, they lack the health knowledge to plan the health sector, while those who have the health knowledge lack the economic skills. Some way must be found to bridge this no man's land and give each an understanding of the thinking of the other. A further reason is the lack of data to make a comprehensive description of the current situation if the plan was to look beyond the activities of the ministry of health and cover all the health sector, public and private, whatever public or private agency was providing it or paying for it. A map is clearly needed if the future path is to be plotted. But such a map has often never been constructed and ministries of health hesitate to go beyond their current area of responsibility and pry into that of others.

How to make a plan

Financial planning consists of six steps:

Step 1 – Establish a base line

The first step is to establish what was spent in the last few years for which data can be collected, how much was spent on what and how it was financed. This means that the precise definition of the health sector has to be established in the local situation.

In the case of the health services, expenditure can be analysed in a number of different ways, as set out in chapter 6. This may involve collecting data which has never been collected before because the accounting system was not designed to yield this type of information. Central is an analysis by source of funds and types of provider. A second analysis is needed by level of service – central services, tertiary hospitals, secondary hospitals and primary care. Third, an analysis is needed to see how much is spent per head in different regions of the country using census data. These three analyses may well point up the changes which need to be made, if higher priority is to be given to primary care and greater equity is to be achieved. More difficult is a breakdown of expenditure by curative (including rehabilitation) and preventive areas, as services at the primary level should be closely integrated. It is not suggested that precise figures should be calculated but that estimates should be attempted. Methods of doing this are set out in the WHO manual mentioned earlier (Mach and Abel-Smith 1983)[1].

In the process of collecting the data and analysing it, an assessment can be made of the efficiency with which existing resources are used.

Is there room for savings by reallocating labour to meet new priorities, by strengthening the supply system to reduce leaks, or by increasing output within existing resources?

Step 2 – Cost a present plan or make a new costed plan

If a 'bottom up' approach to planning has already been introduced, a national plan can be made by adding together and costing the plans coming up from the lower levels of the health system, provided they reflect national guidelines. If there is only a paper setting out the government's broad strategy, this needs to be turned into a costed plan. But there is a preliminary stage of facing up to the question of whether existing services are fully financed. Have the services sufficient resources to fulfil the present functions intended for them? Has the maintenance of buildings been regularly postponed? Is equipment no longer in functioning condition? Are supplies adequate for the services to fulfil their allotted functions in terms of supplies, particularly of drugs? Are there enough functioning vehicles and petrol for the vital tasks of local supervision to be undertaken and for health education programmes to be taken to schools and local meetings? Have the salaries of staff fallen so low that it is unreasonable to expect them to devote their whole time to the services?

If there is a serious problem of under-finance, this has to be quantified. How much extra would be needed to make good the deficiencies and make the services function as intended with expenditures on building maintenance and the renewal of equipment spread over (say) five years? This should clearly be an important objective of any health plan for the future. One way of quantifying the gap is to compare current expenditures in real terms with the level of expenditure when the services were last able to function as intended, with allowance for the running costs of any further health units brought into commission during this time period.

The second stage consists in making the broad national strategy for health development more precise. How much is it desired to spend on what? This means, for example, deciding at what rate the shift to primary care is be made, or the shift to greater geographical equity, or how much is to be devoted to new priorities. The costing should include all capital projects which have been approved and their financial consequences for both capital and current costs. It should also include those promised, even though a time frame has never been given for their completion, because the minister is bound to come under pressure to honour such commitments. It is better to face up to what could and could not be afforded at an early stage before rash promises are made which cannot be fulfilled.

Step 3 – Project likely yield of existing sources of finance

The sources should include both the public sector and the private sector. This is where alternative scenarios can be introduced. A starting point may be the government's economic plan and its projection of economic growth. A safe assumption is that public finance for the health sector will remain the same proportion of the planned gross domestic product in the future as in the past. Experience of a large number of countries suggests that major changes in this relationship are rare and are most likely to occur only with a really radical change in the ideology of the government or when a country is experiencing very rapid economic growth. But national plans always tend to be over-optimistic. They represent what is potentially achievable rather than what is most likely to achieved. Thus one scenario should be based on the assumption that growth is only about half that of the past five years or, if this is lower, about half the rate officially projected. If more money becomes available, the money can be allocated proportionately to make up part of the difference between what was originally planned and what was found to be affordable. This is one advantage of having a plan

Where there already is a compulsory health insurance scheme, the projection should allow for any planned expansion of coverage and for the growth of the employed population.

In the private sector, the easiest assumption is that it will follow the same trend as that sector. But a check can be made on the relative relationships over the past five years. If the public sector has been less and less able to meet the needs of the population, the private sector has probably been increasing its role – particularly if there has been a growth of private hospitals or of unemployed or underemployed doctors. This trend is likely to continue, if policies remain unchanged, at least in the shorter period. If economic growth has been greater than expenditure on public health services over the past five years, again it is likely that the role of the private sector has been increasing and will continue to do so. Projections might be made using different approaches and the most likely prospect selected, allowing for any effects from the growth of the public sector on the likely demands made by patients on that sector.

Step 4 – Quantify any gap between the cost of the present plan and the yield of existing sources of finance

At this stage the minister may wish to report this situation to his or her colleagues in the hope of persuading them to make some firm commitment to put more money into the health sector at the expense of other sectors or by raising taxes, though in most developing countries the scope for the latter is limited.

Step 5 – Explore possibilities for further sources of finance

This is the creative stage. Can ways be found of filling the gap? The first question to be asked is whether all ways have been used of transferring costs to the private sector (such as the costs of industrial and vehicle injuries)? The second question is whether the maximum revenue is being collected from charges which do not fall on the poor (such as private bed charges and charges for immunisation for those going abroad). The third question is whether there are ways of marketing the public services for those willing to pay by establishing pay clinics for medical and dental treatment out of normal working hours.

The fourth question is whether there is a case for introducing or increasing user charges. If this were done, how difficult would it be to exempt the poor? The case may well rest on how under-financed the services are at present and what would be the consequences. Are even poor people being forced to use the private sector to get their important needs met? Has the practice of tipping health staff developed and is it pervasive, with the obvious disadvantages to the poor. If either is the case, there would be an unassailable case for introducing or increasing user charges. If these will enable the public sector to be adequately stocked with drugs, this may attract back patients who have felt forced to find the money to use the private sector. This would need to be fed back into the costed plan.

Beyond this, there is the case for charging full cost to those who bypass the primary care services. To operate this system, it may be necessary to strengthen the urban primary health care system as a first priority.

Next is the question of whether there is a case for promoting systems of voluntary prepayment. Are there agricultural co-operatives which could finance local services by deducting a small percentage from the purchase price of the crops it buys? Can the load be taken off the public health services by developing revolving drug funds?

Finally, is a compulsory health insurance scheme feasible for those in regular employment. How many persons would be covered with their dependants? Can attractive services be devised? Is there the work-force to operate it without damaging the public services? Could such a scheme be affordable by employers and employees? How far would it relieve the public health services of costs or bring in revenue after allowing for its administrative costs?

The gain to the public health services in revenue collected or costs saved from all the above measures found to be practicable need to be brought together and quantified and presented by time period. Compulsory health insurance will take several years to establish. Some charges can be expected to bring in revenue in the short period and others in a longer period.

Step 6 – Reconcile income and expenditure

When all possible sources of extra revenue or transfers of costs have been quantified, this is then compared year by year with planned expenditure and any gap is identified. Have any ways been found of increasing efficiency and redeploying resources? Is there room for using less advanced technology and how much could be saved if this were done? Is there any reason to expect that foreign donors will contribute either to the costs of administering charges or some new policy developments included in the plan? Helping countries establish new sources of finance is a potentially attractive proposition for donors, partly because the expenditure is once and for all and partly because it assists the country to become more self-reliant in the future.

If, after all possibilities have been explored, a gap still remains, means must be found of closing it. Some hoped-for developments may have to be cut out of the plan. Some way may have to be found to reduce the costs of the tertiary hospitals. At the very least they must have tough resource limits placed on them to contain growth which is demand-led. The strengthening of primary care should enable their role to be reduced. It may be possible to close some hospitals or parts of hospitals where occupancy rates are low and there is over-provision relative to available resources. It may be necessary to increase the distance rural people will have to travel to reach facilities. Or it may be necessary to rethink the whole mix of different grades of personnel on which the existing structure of services is based. It may be necessary to develop a long-term plan to use less highly qualified staff and make greater use of auxiliaries. This will have major implications for future training programmes and the financial consequences will need to be worked back into a revised plan.

In general a decision to make real cuts in a service's expenditure will depend on a number of factors, the likely impact of the financial squeezer, the anticipated political reaction, the likely impact in health terms and the opportunities in the service for making real efficiency savings' (Segall 1991: p. 56)[2].

Why a long-term plan?

Partly because of the possible need to re-gear the mix of personnel needed to provide services, a plan needs to look well into the future – for a period of some 15 to 20 years. But it should also be recognised that the running cost of any additional hospital beds must determine how many extra beds can be afforded. While the first five years may be thought through in depth, the remaining 10 or more years may be only sketched in outline. But thinking over a longer period is necessary simply because it takes so long to build major hospitals and not only to train different categories of staff but also to accumulate a sufficient stock to run the services. Any major redeployment of resources, which is seen as too painful or politically contentious if carried out over a short period, may be more acceptable if phased over a long period. For example, it is easier to retrain staff or not replace staff on retirement than simply make them redundant.

The process of financial planning obliges countries to confront painful alternatives. Some possible options, such as charging for services, will inevitably be politically unpopular. Similarly, a decision to cut down on what has been planned, for example, by postponing promised hospital developments, will also be unpopular among certain groups of the population. On the other hand, to abandon the political stance that there is a real intention to bring primary health care within reach of the whole population would be politically unpopular among other sections of the population.

It is because the choices can be painful that some countries drift on from year to year with short-term plans, responding to the noisiest pressures, and waiting for some extraordinary donor or economic miracle to get them off the horns of these dilemmas. Each year the timetable for achieving 'Health for All' is thus tacitly put back, though never openly abandoned. This may have been inevitable in countries faced with all the vagaries of the economic crisis. But in some countries there may have been a lack of political will to embark on any form of resolute action which will take them where they are pledged to go.

Some examples of completed financial plans

The Netherlands

The plan allowed for a growth of health expenditure (public and private) in the period 1986 to 2000 of only 1.2 per cent, which was almost entirely due to changes in morbidity as a result of the aging population. This meant that the share of health care in the gross national product would actually fall from 8.3 per cent in 1986 to 7.8 per cent in the year 2000. A growth of 1.9 per cent per year in expenditure on primary health care was to be balanced by a decline in expenditure on hospital care.

Sweden

The plan envisaged a near doubling of expenditure on primary care between 1985 and 2000. Expenditure on secondary and tertiary care would fall from 73 per cent of health expenditure in 1985 to 61 per cent in the year 2000. Despite the aging of the population, it was calculated that health expenditure would only have to increase from 7.8 per cent of the gross domestic product in 1985 to 8.0 per cent in the year 2000.

Costa Rica

The plan envisaged the completion of the process of integrating the preventive and curative services in combined health centres, the development of a personal doctor system within primary care, and the rebuilding of some hospitals, which would require extra recurrent costs. It was calculated that the cost could be contained within the likely yield of compulsory health insurance contributions by the year 1990 when their 'Health for All' programme would be completed.

Zimbabwe

The financial plan was built up in five stages. The first was to cost the requirements for capital construction, mainly needed to rebuild the primary health facilities which were greatly damaged during the war of independence. The second was to calculate the recurrent costs arising out of these developments and the training programme needed to meet the additional staff requirements. The third step was to cost any actions specified in the detailed plan of action which were not included in the above. The fourth step was to project revenue on the cautious assumption that the same proportion of the gross domestic product would be spent on health services in the year 2000 as in 1985. The final step was to examine the potential revenue from introducing a compulsory health insurance scheme.

On these assumptions it was calculated that health sector spending would need to grow by 80 per cent by the year 2000: 90 per cent of the extra expenditure would be on primary health care. It was found that both the expansion of the health services and the planned water and sanitation programme could be contained, without any increase in the proportion of the gross domestic product devoted to the health sector. Any shortfall could be absorbed by the potential yield of health insurance contributions.

Conclusion

The message of this chapter can be simply summarised. No plan is realistic until it is costed: it amounts to no more than a dream. Second, a modest plan is safer than an ambitious plan. It is easier to add to a plan later on than cut it back, Third, planning expenditure without at the same time planning revenue is no more than window-shopping. A way has to be found to balance future expenditure with future revenue. A long-term plan is needed:

- to make sure that primary health care really can be made accessible to the whole population;
- to avoid training people who cannot make a living in the public or private sectors;

- to prevent building what cannot be staffed and maintained;
- to provide for a gradual shift to new priorities, to greater geographical equity and, if necessary, to a different mix of personnel.

Notes

1 Mach, E. and Abel-Smith, B. (1983), *Planning the Finances of the Health Sector; a Manual for Developing Countries*, WHO, Geneva.
2 Segall, M. (1991), 'Health sector planning led by management of recurrent expenditure: an agenda for action-research', *Health Policy and Planning*.

INDEX

accidents
  industrial, 23, 29, 54, 164–5
  road traffic, 38, 52, 54–5, 165–6
advertising
  alcohol, 43–4
  drugs, 122, 125–7
  and health promotion, 40–1, 43–4
  tobacco, 38, 43–4, 59
age, and mortality, 6
  see also demographic change;
    elderly
agricultural policy, 49–50, 51
aid for developing countries, 136,
    155, 158, 159, 174, 226
  see also loans
AIDS
  expenditure, 154–5, 159
  health promotion, 35
alcohol
  advertising, 43–4
  consumption, 28, 36, 38, 39, 52
allopathic medicine, 34
Alma Ata conference, 107
auxiliaries, 100

beliefs *see* values and beliefs
birth rate, 15
Bismark, O., and compulsory health
    insurance, 71
Black Report, 21, 24
Blaxter, M., 5
budgets
  GPs, 214
  hospital, 198–9, 204–5
  regulation of, 86
  staff, 113–15
  see also financing

cancer, 9
capitation payments, 69–70, 197–8,
    216

Catholic control of hospitals, 66,
    67–8
Centre for Development Studies
    (CENDES), 81–2, 115
charges *see* user charges
charitable hospitals, 66–7
children's health, 8, 43, 44, 50, 55
  see also infant mortality
classification
  hospital, 140–2
  occupational, 21–2, 24–5
co-payment, 196
  see also user charges
Cochrane, A., 9
community financing, 173–5
community health workers, 111, 113
community participation, 110–11
comparative approach to studying
    health, 5, 8–16
competition in health care, 186, 210,
    213–16
compulsory health insurance
  advantages and disadvantages,
      178–9
  in Britain, 71
  in Chile, 179
  and demand, 154
  equity, 179–80
  in Germany, 70–1
  history, 70–3
  organisation, 183–4
  practicability, 181–3, 225
  service provision, 107, 185–8
  transition to universal care, 73–6
consumer choice *see* competition
consumer demand, control of, 160
  see also community financing; user
      charges
consumer movement, 128
consumer participation, 110–11
continuity of care